# NEO
# SOUL

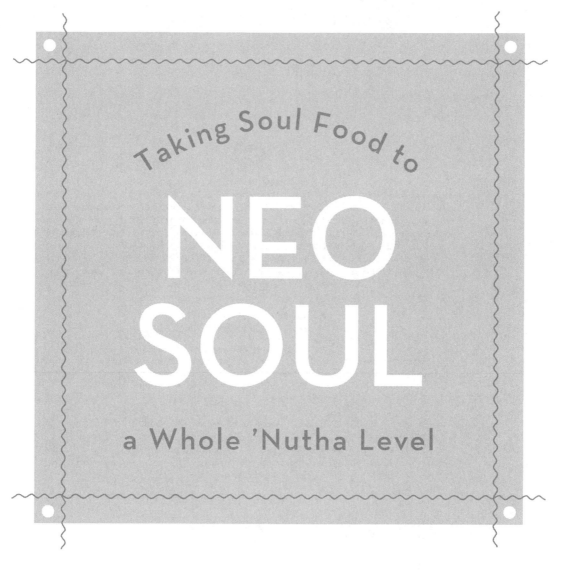

Taking Soul Food to

# NEO SOUL

## a Whole 'Nutha Level

# LINDSEY WILLIAMS

Foreword by Sylvia Woods,
owner of Harlem's world-famous restaurant Sylvia's

AVERY • *a member of Penguin Group (USA) Inc.* • *New York*

Published by the Penguin Group

Penguin Group (USA) Inc., 375 Hudson Street, New York, New York 10014, USA • Penguin Group
(Canada), 90 Eglinton Avenue, Suite 700, Toronto, Ontario M4P 2Y3, Canada (a division of Pearson
Penguin Canada Inc.) • Penguin Books Ltd, 80 Strand, London WC2R 0RL, England • Penguin
Ireland, 25 St Stephen's Green, Dublin 2, Ireland (a division of Penguin Books Ltd) • Penguin Group
(Australia), 250 Camberwell Road, Camberwell, Victoria 3124, Australia (a division of Pearson
Australia Group Pty Ltd) • Penguin Books India Pvt Ltd, 11 Community Centre, Panchsheel Park,
New Delhi–110 017, India • Penguin Group (NZ), Cnr Airborne and Rosedale Roads, Albany,
Auckland 1310, New Zealand (a division of Pearson New Zealand Ltd) • Penguin Books
(South Africa) (Pty) Ltd, 24 Sturdee Avenue, Rosebank, Johannesburg 2196, South Africa

Penguin Books Ltd, Registered Offices:
80 Strand, London WC2R 0RL, England

Interior photographs reprinted courtesy of the author.
The following recipes are original creations submitted by Brenda L. Jenkins: Banana Bread (page 37);
B.J.'s Potato Salad (page 65); Cole Slaw (page 67); Cornbread Stuffing (page 78); Bread Pudding
(page 145); Fried Apples (page 148); Peach Cobbler (page 149); Blueberry Buckle (page 150);
and Pumpkin Pie (page 152).

ISBN 1-58333-194-8

Printed in the United States of America

*Book design by Stephanie Huntwork*

*Neo Soul* is dedicated to my grandfather, Herbert Woods (1925-2001), a man who loved me, taught me, and understood me.

And to my father, who died before I knew him.

# Acknowledgments

When I was interviewing chefs, I found that many talented African-American chefs didn't do soul food, as if soul food were beneath them. Leroy Ian Charles is one of the best chefs I've ever met, and he specializes not only in soul food, but also in Caribbean and vegetarian dishes. Leroy's influence is present throughout the book. Brenda L. Jenkins, a superb chef, helped me create many of the *Neo Soul* recipes. I would also like to give a special thanks to Nesley Watson for all his help; and to my nutritionist, Alicia Flynn, thank you. Writer Neeraja Viswanathan was there when I needed her and delivered excellent work in record-breaking time. Photographer Ronnie Wright is one of the best, and I'm honored to include some of his work. The emphasis in *Neo Soul* is on healthy, flavorful eating, while trying to keep the tradition of soul food alive, and all of them contributed their expertise.

Megan Newman and Lissa Brown at Avery offered enthusiasm and know-how. Thank you to everyone at Avery for believing in *Neo Soul*.

The professionals at LifeTime Media had my back, held my hand, and contributed enormously to *Neo Soul*. Thank you to Jacqueline Grace and her staff. Most of all, thank you to Cathy Repetti, editor, adviser, and now friend.

Thank you to everyone who contributed in some way to my crazy life:

Mom, for teaching me never to settle and to keep my eye on the prize; Grandma, for the foundation you gave me and for being so tough yet always there no matter what; to my sister, Tamicka, and niece, Zaire—you are the best; all the Woods and Williams aunts and uncles and cousins, you are a great family.

To Russell Simmons, thank you for giving me my first job; Bill Steffany, you're a great friend and you've taught me a lot. Big shout-out to the original ten people at Def Jam & Rush at 298 Elizabeth St. We had some great experiences; nothing can duplicate them. Walter Dawkins, my homey, you've been down with me a long time; thank you for everything you've done for me (I owe you); thank you, Charles Koppleman, for teaching me how to make money in a crazy business and for giving me such great opportunities at EMI; Daniel Glass, thank you for the experience; Marcus Morton, no matter what, you're my homey, kid; thank you to Mia Young, Beverly, and all the reps and friends. Thank you, Gary Beech, for all your support, and Ken Wilson for the years of friendship.

To all the artists I worked with in the past: LL Cool J, Public Enemy (Chuck and Flav); and Speech from Arrested Development; Slick Rick (Stand Up). And a shout-out to Bill Adler.

Thanks as well go to all my friends who contributed recipes. Drew Nieporent from Nobu, John Byrne from Scarborough Fair, Gabriel of

Gabriel's, and Heather Bryant—I appreciate all of your knowledge and support.

Shout-outs to Harlem and Lenox Avenue; all my clients, especially at the Apollo Theater, *All My Children* (John Baxley), Mark and Kelly Ripa, VH-1, MTV, LA Reid and family, Latrell Sprewell and family; everybody from Noble Avenue in the Bronx; Puff, Flex (I see you—you killin' them), and Chris Littie . . . these are the guys who took the game to the next level; to Wendy Williams—I read your book and it was amazing; Jam Master Jay and Easy E—you're both missed by many; Londell McMillan and Firm; Iris and Bob Egan; Raquel Gordian and family; Chrissy and Cheryl; Lindsay Stern; Reebok Sports Club, where it all started; and the Natural Cooking School; Roslyn Burns; Inez Cain and Laura Beatty; Raymond McGuire, Reggie Osia and family; the Bradley family and J.B.; Nelson George, who got me on the basketball court when I was 300 pounds; Philip Wong and all my catering staff; a big thanks to all my vendors; Jim Thaller of ABF Consulting, for helping me to keep my life straight; Karu Daniels and all of the other journalists who have taken a real interest in my story; my hometown of Hemingway, South Carolina, for giving me that Southern foundation; and to all my friends who I forgot—peace, be seein' ya; thank you, Reverend Calvin Butts, my pastor, at Abyssinian Baptist Church.

I thank God for all of the great opportunities I've had and for bringing Dara Stewart, my editor, into my life. She has been kind and patient, but most of all, an advocate extraordinaire for *Neo Soul* from day one.

And finally, my thanks to Harry Fobbs,
the best A&R guy in the business
and a true hip-hopper forever.

# Contents

# Foreword

When we opened up Sylvia's Soul Food Restaurant in 1962, we knew it was going to be a family business. My grandkids were just babies—some weren't even born yet—but they were already growing up in the restaurant business. Everyone had a job, including Lindsey. At first, I used to put him to work cleaning the floors and washing dishes, but he hated those jobs. Lindsey is the kind of person who wants to be out front, greeting the customers and making sure everyone is having a good time.

It wasn't easy for him growing up. He was born a chubby kid, and as he grew older, he just grew heavier and heavier. I remember him not being able to tie his own shoes because he couldn't bend down, or straining to do sit-ups. I used to feel so bad for him, because I struggled with my own weight issues when I was younger, and I'd see people in the restaurant who always had to have seconds—even though they knew they shouldn't. His mother and I tried everything we knew of back then to help him lose weight, and I know he tried a lot of things himself. But nothing seemed to work, and it broke my heart, because he was such a good, cheerful child.

When he was working in the record business, he put on so much weight that the situation became critical. I was worried about the stress he was under. I think that situation, and finally dealing openly with his weight issue, was what allowed him to lose the weight. Now he's doing just beautifully, and I pray that he never has to go back to the weight he once was.

Lindsey has brought a lot to Sylvia's Restaurant. In addition to taking pressure off his mother for the catering, he's come up with a lot of great ideas about the food and how to attract new customers. We've been in business for forty-two years, and we just never thought too much about serving baked chicken instead of fried chicken, or trying to make our foods healthier. Now, with Lindsey, these are things that we're thinking about for the very first time. Lindsey has a lot of suggestions, and being a natural people person, he really gets people to listen.

I think it's a wonderful idea to make soul food more accessible to people who want to eat healthy and watch their weight. When you've struggled as much as Lindsey, it's important to share your experiences and your discoveries with the whole world. Soul food is just food cooked with a lot of love, and everyone should be able to eat it. I know that's what this cookbook is about, and that you'll enjoy the recipes inside.

—Sylvia Woods

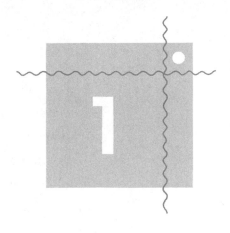

# My Story

My name is Lindsey Williams and I'm an addict.

I'm not the kind of addict you think I am. For many people, the word *addict* means something sleazy and illegal. But I don't use drugs, and I'm not an alcoholic. I am addicted to food. I am particularly addicted to flour and sugar, but in general I'm just addicted to food. What does this mean? It means that while so-called "normal" people can eat a bag of potato chips, I can't. If I eat one chip, then I'll have to have another. And another. I'll eat bags and bags of chips, and I won't be able to stop—even if I'm not hungry. My being a food addict means that my eating habits are beyond my control. I've been this way as long as I can remember, but it took me years to admit it to myself.

My troubles with food haunted me for most of my life, to the point that I truly believed I was the only person with such an overwhelming addiction.

I was obese, and that made me feel like the freak of my family. I shopped at special stores for my extra-large clothes. I was always meeting with doctors. I was always hungry.

By the age of twenty-six, I had a very successful career in the music industry, working with some of the greatest rap artists of all time. I had a loving family and a beautiful wife. But the defining factor of my life was my battle with my weight and dealing with a food addiction I didn't know I had.

# GRANDMA, THE QUEEN OF SOUL FOOD

When I was growing up, everyone watched what I ate, and there was always a list of foods that weren't allowed on my plate. Good foods, too, like macaroni and cheese, fried chicken, cheese grits. The problem was that, in my family, those foods were everywhere. It was soul food, and it was the way my family had made a living for three generations.

You see, my grandmother, Sylvia Woods, is the Queen of Soul Food. Her Harlem restaurant, Sylvia's, has recently celebrated its forty-second anniversary. Music moguls, movie stars, star athletes, and a former U.S. president frequent the restaurant to sample my grandmother's world-famous recipes for soul food. The restaurant began as a humble one-counter luncheonette in 1962 and now occupies a full block in Harlem. My grandmother has recently expanded even further, marketing her special brand of soul food in supermarkets all across the country—everything from canned collard greens to black-eyed pea soup to her very special hot sauce. She even opened up a sister restaurant in Atlanta. Virtually every member of my family was involved, or is still involved, in the family business.

You can see my dilemma. Here was the rich, flavorful history of my grandmother's restaurant. You can call it soul food, comfort food, or Southern cooking—but for me it was just the way we cooked, and it is the best food in the world. Nothing compares to marinated spare ribs covered in barbecue sauce, with sides of fried okra, candied yams, and fresh golden cornbread. My grandmother always said that soul food was just Southern food cooked with a lot of soul and love, and everyone who stepped into her restaurant could tell that this was true.

And then there was me, the fat kid.

I didn't know I was an addict then. According to everyone I knew, I was the kid who stuck out, who ate too much, who had a "weight problem." All that food in the restaurant was only for the customers; I was on a different diet. Many different diets, in fact. The only problem was that they never seemed to work—well, not for very long, anyway.

While the whole family made its living from soul food, I was struggling. I was usually hungry, but even when I wasn't I was picking at food—out of boredom, stress, or depression. On Sunday mornings, my mother would make breakfast, but I couldn't even wait until it was served. I stuffed my face with doughnuts and cookies and then sat down with my family for a big Sunday breakfast. My mother eventually enrolled me in an obesity research program at Mount Sinai Hospital in New York City. I was pulled out of school and lived at the hospital for nearly five months. The hospital food, of course, was horrible, so when my friends visited, I asked them to bring some Snickers. I lost weight—but it didn't take me long to put it back on again. In my last year of high school, I went to a weight-loss center in North Carolina called Structure House where the focus is on weight loss and discovering new, healthier foods. But Structure House did not discuss food addiction, so the program didn't have lasting benefits for me. Still, over the next two decades I would be in and out of Structure House, battling myself as my weight yo-yoed up and down.

Did this get me down? Definitely. Anyone with a weight problem will tell you that being the obese kid in school was pretty awful. I never got used to nicknames like "Fat Albert," and being teased when I couldn't run quickly. It was upsetting, and my way of dealing with it was to hide my feelings and put on a happy front. I wanted to convince people that I was just a normal, fun-loving kid, despite being obese. As for the eating—that was my secret. I was a closet eater, and closet eaters don't eat in public. We like to sneak the food when no one is looking, thinking that if we're not caught, then we're not really eating.

## THE PERILOUS YEARS IN CORPORATE AMERICA

I had big plans for myself. I grew up loving all kinds of music, but rap was special. In the late seventies, rap wasn't played on the radio or on MTV—you only heard it on the streets. Some of the greatest rappers around came from my neighborhood, and they were local heroes. Even from an early age, I always knew that I wanted to be in the music industry, but it was only after high school that I realized I wanted to be an executive, not an artist. And I knew that there was just one job for me: at Def Jam Recordings, with Russell Simmons.

I was working as an intern at another record label, but I often pestered Russell about a job when he came into Sylvia's. One fateful day, he finally said, "Come see me tomorrow at 9:30." That very day, Russell put me to work with Bill Stephany, who was head of promotions. I knew I had to prove myself. I learned the names and positions of everyone at every

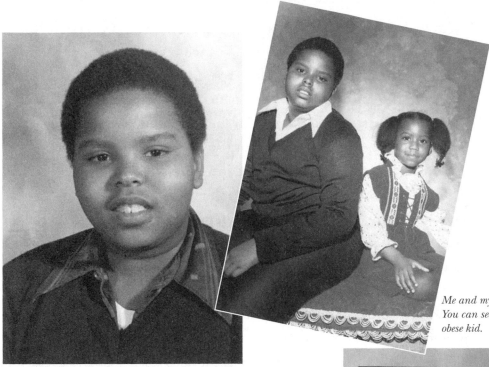

Me and my sister, Tamicka.
You can see I'm already an
obese kid.

*At twelve, the junk food has taken its toll.*

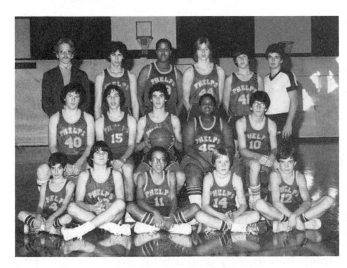

*At boarding school, I tried to be athletic and find ways to get into
some kind of shape. I even played on the basketball team. I had a
good time, but this wasn't the way to permanent weight loss and
healthy eating. That's me, second from the right in the middle row.*

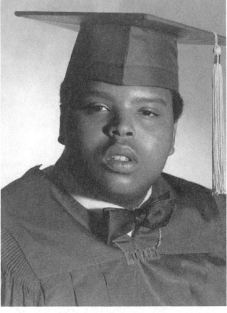

*At eighteen, I was unhealthy and obese, graduating from high school and dreaming of making it in
the music business.*

radio station in town, and I was able to show Bill that I was serious about the business. Eventually, Bill became one of my closest friends.

The harder I worked, the more responsibilities I was given. Soon I started going on tour with the acts as the tour promotion manager. Before the artists arrived in each city, I made sure that the radio stations were playing their singles, the record stores were promoting them, and the concert venues were decked out and expecting us. It was a wild, hectic time. Tours were always crazy, and as the venues got bigger and bigger, so did the problems. I had to deal with groupies and catfights, egos and drunken brawls. As wild as things got, though, I still loved the business and the music.

But the rap business wasn't the best way to stay healthy. My weight went up and down as I got more immersed in the crazy life of a rap music promoter. I didn't think too much about my health or my emotional well-being. To make matters worse, I was also a total perfectionist. Whenever something went wrong, I thought it was my fault—my fault that the shows weren't selling, my fault that the stations weren't playing us, my fault the artists weren't getting along. It was all spiraling out of control. Even though Def Jam was becoming the hottest record company in the business, and even though any young rap fan would've given his right arm for my job, I was wondering if there was something else out there for me.

In 1991, the head of rap music at Chrysalis left the company. The next thing I knew, I was offered the job. Soon after that, EMI Records took over.

This was what I had been waiting for my whole life. This was the big job, the one where I'd be part of a nationwide production company with unlimited resources, and the ability to attract virtually any artist into its fold. The job paid extremely well, it was prestigious, and I thought that all my dreams were coming true. To the casual observer, I had everything: a high profile, a

*Here I am at nineteen years old at Structure House with my mom. I've actually lost weight at this point.*

*The Williams men at the first Million Man March in Washington, D.C. Left to right: Uncle Kenneth, Grandfather Herbert, Uncle Van, Cousin Che, and me.*

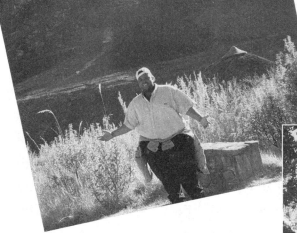

*Here I am on location in South Africa, shooting a video with Arrested Development. I'm getting close to my record weight—and I'm giving that mountain some competition for the biggest thing in the photo.*

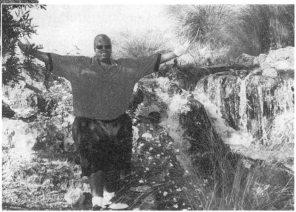

*In 1995, I attended the PGA in Palm Beach, Florida. I seem to be having a good time, but believe me, I was sick.*

high-paying job in the record industry, a beautiful wife, luxury cars, a big house, and cash in my pocket.

But I wasn't taking care of myself or my family. And the record business was changing. Suddenly artists were demanding a Rolex before they would sign with you. They wanted more money, more exposure. I had to face the fact that my love for the industry was gone. Also, my marriage was falling apart. I started gaining weight at a rate that was staggering, even to me. Suddenly I was 350 pounds, and I was only 5'5". I had stopped any pretense of going to the gym. I ate compulsively, even when I wasn't hungry. I poured all my energy into work and eating, even though neither one meant much to me anymore.

## HITTING ROCK BOTTOM

The turning point wasn't something I did, it was something God did. When EMI Records folded, I started a fledgling label with an investment banker friend. I hadn't saved any money and I had huge bills to pay off. Then, on New Year's Day 1997, everything came crashing down. On that day, my wife told me she was leaving. I couldn't comprehend it, until she packed up her bags and actually left the house. Three days later, I got a letter from my investment banker friend stating that he no longer wanted to start the label and had removed the funds. I had gone from being a vice president of a prestigious music corporation to being unemployed and unmarried—in a matter of a couple of months.

I was also 400 pounds, more than I'd ever weighed before.

I began to isolate myself, suffering from massive depression. I couldn't get out of bed. I couldn't stop crying. All I did was eat, and compulsively, even when I stopped tasting the food. My family and friends were worried

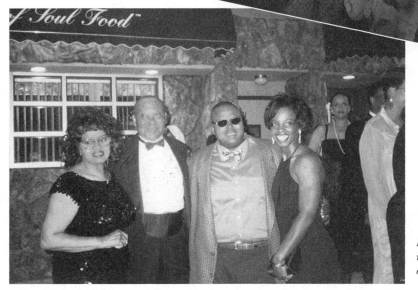

*On vacation in Barbados in 1996.*

*Me and Mom celebrating Sylvia's "Queen of Soul Food" anniversary in 1997.*

*In front of Sylvia's that night with my grandparents and my ex-wife, Jaena.*

sick about me, but I couldn't even begin to understand what they were feeling. I couldn't believe I had let everything slip through my fingers. To make matters worse, I had no money. I sold my house and my cars and moved into my mother's basement. I certainly didn't have any money for Structure House.

Then an old friend came to visit. After listening to me for a while, she asked me to come to a support group. I'd gone with her a couple of times before and had never felt very comfortable. But I didn't know what else to do. At the meeting, I listened to what the others were saying. And for the first time, I realized that I wasn't alone. There were other people struggling out there with weight problems, with compulsive eating, and with food addiction. Suddenly, *addict* wasn't a dirty word anymore.

I realized that obesity was a problem that many people had and suffered with quietly, without talking about it. It didn't make me weird or different. I believe that many obese people suffer from a food addiction and just don't know it. Food addicts are surrounded by misinformation, by prejudices, and by conflicting advice. Nobody had told them that it was a disorder—certainly, no one had told me. Now, going to support groups, it felt like there was light at the end of the tunnel. I could see the way out.

## STARTING FROM SCRATCH . . . AND FINDING MY WAY

Working out was hard. At first, I couldn't even do the simplest cardio; I was too out of shape to do anything but a very low-impact workout. But I set small goals for myself and tried to be patient. When I wasn't at the gym, I was going to meetings and learning more and more about my addiction. The support group was a place to find companion-ship and answers. And without my family, I could never have started on the path to recovery and rejoining society. I felt that I was on a spiritual path, and even went to church every Sunday. It was the first time I really took care of my total self.

And yes, I was losing weight. I realized that I didn't have control over my food addiction, and the best thing I could do was deal with the issues as they came up. I knew what was good for me, and I knew what foods I needed to avoid. I started slow with the exercise and set goals for myself. Gradually, I got into better shape and I began to see a difference. I restricted myself to three healthy meals a day, with no snacking. Was I hungry? Sure I was. In fact, for the first three months I was starving. But then I began to see a difference in my body, and that felt more important, more exciting, than not being hungry.

It took a long time to drop the weight, but I did it. Eventually, I went from 400 pounds to 160 pounds.

## COMING HOME: CATERING AND A CAREER IN FOOD

Now that I had reconnected with my life, I found myself thinking about my future. I had been part of the music industry for nearly fif-teen years, and I wasn't sure I knew how to do anything else. But I didn't feel that the record business was fun anymore, and I now wanted to have a good time at whatever I did. By 1999, I was working as a manager at Sylvia's. You would have thought working at the restaurant was hard when you're trying to lose weight, but actually I was enjoying myself. I brought my own food to the restaurant, and I was working on issues that had nothing to do with fried chicken. Besides, I realized that I enjoyed being out in front, greeting people and watching them have a good time. There was something immensely satisfying about watching people eating great food in a lively atmosphere.

As I became more social, I began to spend summers at the Hamptons with friends. One of them owned a popular club named Rocco's. We were chatting one day, and I offered to set up a "gospel brunch" for an upcoming Sunday. A gospel brunch is a Sylvia's special—soul food, friendly caterers, a great setting, and to top it all off, a gospel choir that performed during the buffet. It was my first independent project, and everything went perfectly. What started out as a onetime deal for a hundred people became an immensely popular Sunday institution at Rocco's for three hundred people. I spent all summer setting up gospel brunches in the Hamptons, and when I came back, I knew what I wanted to do with my life. I started Lindsey Catering 125 in the fall of 2001.

## THE BIRTH OF NEO-SOUL FOOD

I knew that Sylvia's Catering, run by my mother, was doing very well, and by her side I received an education in the business of preparing, serving, and creating delicious Southern meals. But I was ready to do something a little different. My goal was to enhance the soul food experience, give it an edge, and make it more chic. My sense was that most people thought of soul food—Southern food in general—as homey and comforting, but also unsophisticated and cheap. I believed that if it could be prepared and presented elegantly, people would be more likely to respect and appreciate the business of soul food. Most important, people associated soul food with unhealthy cooking, a cuisine that was high in fat and cholesterol. In short, it was something you ate around the house informally.

And that's how I got the idea for Neo-Soul Food.

At Lindsey Catering 125, we upgraded the décor and the presentation of the food so that you really knew you were having an exciting upscale dining experience. We also experimented with a variety of ingredients and alternative methods of preparation. For example, instead of candied yams, which was a soul food staple, why not a whipped yam soufflé? It tasted just as good but looked far more sophisticated. It was the same comfort food in a new form. Another example is collard greens, which are traditionally cooked in pork grease. We sautéed them in olive oil instead, and chopped them into fine strings so they would be easier to eat, with less risk of a mess. We tried new ways to bring soul food up to date, to make it uptown with a downtown flair. We also used free-range chicken and organic beef. Organic food created the new generation of cooking, and I wanted Lindsey Catering 125 to break new ground in the way people thought of and enjoyed soul food.

And it seemed to be working. Suddenly I was handling a number of projects. Most important, I was working with my main chef, Leroy Ian Charles, to create more and more healthy soul food dishes. Leroy had grown up in the kitchens of Sylvia's Restaurant and had helped me out with my gospel brunches at Rocco's. I'm not sure what it is—his seasonings, his ingredients, his measures—but I believe that he's one of the premier soul food chefs in the country.

Initially, most of my clients were corporations, like Morgan Stanley, looking for an unusual brunch or dinner. We also became the regular caterers for ABC, particularly for soap operas such as *All My Children*. Soon I began going back to my music industry connections. We started with small gigs, like dinners for J Records (which produces Alicia Keys)

# · EXERCISE TIPS ·

Exercise was vital to my weight loss. It required hard work and perseverance. You, too, can begin slowly and build up endurance and strength, and before long you will see positive results.

- EXERCISE TIP #1: GETTING STARTED:

Getting started is largely a matter of attitude. At first I could barely do any exercise at all, but I told myself that I wanted an athletic lifestyle. I took every opportunity that I could to work some form of exercise into my lifestyle. When I began to have knee problems—mostly due to my previous weight—I found it really difficult to do cardio. So I took up swimming, which isn't as hard on the knees. Try to find activities that you like, and see it as a lifestyle change, rather than some chore that you have to do. Once you tell yourself that you're going to live an athletic lifestyle, you'll be looking for opportunities to exercise.

- EXERCISE TIP #2: CARDIOVASCULAR EXERCISE

When I first started working out, I did cardio. I was too big to do anything fast or complicated, so I worked out on the Precor machine, at the lowest level. The most important thing about cardio is to do over 20 minutes, because only then do you start burning fat. The good news is that 30 minutes is usually enough to start seeing results. I started at the lowest level on the Precor machine and stayed there for two weeks, gradually increasing my workout time. With cardio, it's important to set small goals for yourself and steadily increase the challenge.

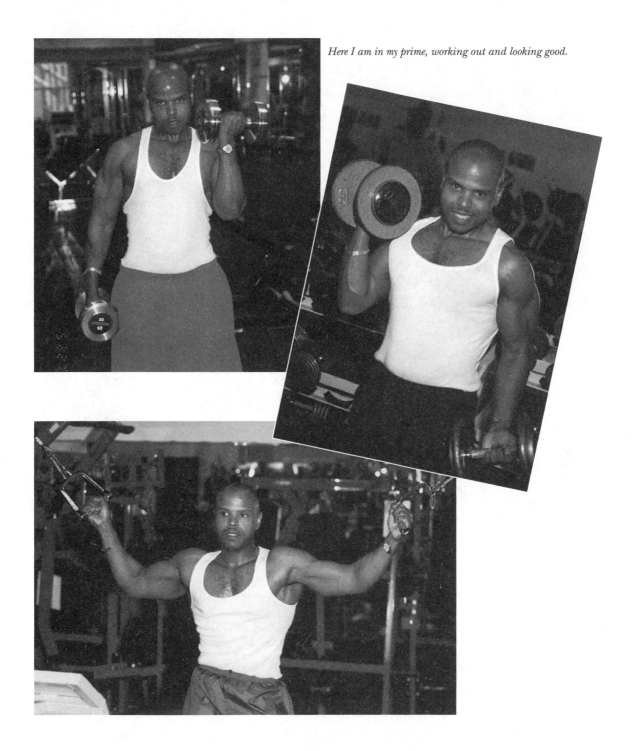

*Here I am in my prime, working out and looking good.*

- EXERCISE TIP #3: WEIGHT TRAINING

Weight training has become more popular, and can help you get definition and muscle tone as you start losing weight. If you're lifting free weights, then you should start with lighter weights and do more reps. The number of reps is what counts. If you're bench pressing, it's extremely important to have someone spotting you so you don't injure yourself. The most important thing about weight training is keeping a good form and posture. For this, it's a good idea to work with a trainer so you know how to maximize results.

- EXERCISE TIP #4: TRAINERS

When you're starting out with your exercise program, it might be a good idea to get a trainer. You don't have to work out with a trainer the whole time, but initially, a trainer can show you how to use the machines and to lift weights with the proper form. My trainer was known as "The Duke," and he taught me the right way to lift weights years ago. Because of that, when I started again, I remembered what he taught me and was able to do them on my own. Trainers are there to tailor the exercise program to your needs, and to encourage you to go to the next level. They're professionals who can help you not only with your exercise routine, but with your diet and general health as well.

and other small companies. Revisiting my old record industry colleagues helped me realize how far I'd come. Because of my weight loss, and my belief in healthy eating, people took Lindsey Catering 125 seriously.

I know that many obese people feel that others are watching and judging them. And sometimes they are. But in my experience, most people are rooting for you to lose the weight, and to be a success. I spent hours at the

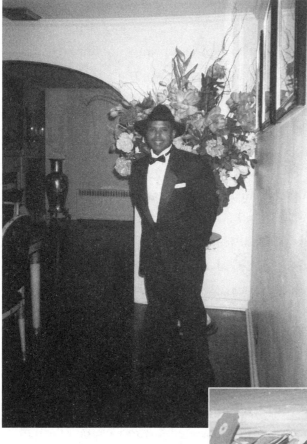

*Slimmed down, healthy, and alive in every sense of the word. It's 2000, and don't I look fine?*

*Two years later, I had put on a bit of the old weight, but at least I was able to look good in a bathing suit.*

Reebok Gym, which is frequented by a large number of celebrity clientele. I was very focused on losing weight, but along the way, I met a lot of people—many famous—who kept my spirits up and encouraged me to continue. Ed Bradley, for example, always came up to me to find out how I was doing. When I started losing weight, Jerry Seinfeld came by and congratulated me. Even celebrities understand the struggle of weight loss, and most people really want you to succeed. And both Russell Simmons and Puff Daddy, my old friends, were amazed at how much I'd lost.

As I lost the weight, people wanted to know how I did it. I appeared on a number of talk shows, including the *Queen Latifah Show* and the *Montel Williams Show*. *People* magazine even featured me in an article. But nothing compared to the day that I got a call from Oprah's producer. I was so nervous—to me, Oprah is like a queen, someone who has achieved enormous success and, of course, struggled with weight loss herself. But she wanted me on her show, and after meeting with her producers, I flew to Chicago. Like everyone else, she wanted to know how I did it. I was happy to tell her, and happy to encourage others to take care of themselves.

As a result of the hard work and the publicity, Lindsey Catering 125 developed a highly visible, celebrity clientele. At the former Manhattan hot spot Chateau, we catered events such as a New Year's Party for Britney Spears and Justin Timberlake in December of 2001. We also did a birthday party for Tori Spelling, and a private party for Paul McCartney and Heather Mills, to celebrate her spread for *Vogue* magazine.

My private chefs worked for a number of high-profile clients, most notably Kelly Ripa and Mark Consuelos, who hired one of my chefs on a regular basis. Latrell Sprewell, who eats organic and healthy, uses one of my chefs every night. We catered the annual gala for the Christopher Wallace Foundation (which had a guest list of more than 450 people). Knicks point guard Stephon Marbury's wedding (which was also over 400 people) kept us busy. Thanks to my record industry connections, we did a lot of back-stage catering, particularly for LL Cool J.

But there were more changes along the way. I merged Lindsey Catering 125 with Sylvia's Catering, and became a percentage partner in the family business. In 2005, my business grew and transformed yet again. My creative juices were boiling over, and simply catering food was no longer enough. I wanted to produce the whole event. That's how Neo Soul Events & Catering was born.

Another goal of mine is to market my own organic soul food line of products. I want to create neo-soul food products made from organic ingredients and with less salt and sugar. I hope to even have frozen or ready-to-cook entrées.

There's a lot more I am going to do with my life, but I know it will take time. In the meantime, things are pretty good. I still deal with my food addiction every day, and I try never to forget that I'm an addict. I meet with my support group and go to my gym and watch what I'm eating. I know I couldn't have done it without my faith in God, and I try to stay close to my spirituality at all times.

## THE COOKBOOK . . . AND HOW SOUL FOOD CAN BE GOOD FOR YOU

This cookbook is part of that plan. In most African-American families, food is a big part of life. Every event, every holiday is centered on food—usually a big buffet with a variety of sides and desserts. With a culture so immersed in entertaining and eating, African-Americans need to watch what they're eating. But many don't.

The traditional African-American diet can be high in sodium and cholesterol and may not include enough fruits or vegetables. Another problem may be the poverty facing many African-Americans. When you're poor, you tend to eat easy, unhealthy food, such as fast food or junk food, simply because it's cheaper and more accessible. Often, African-Americans, especially lower-income ones, haven't learned the importance of a consistent exercise plan. The results of this lifestyle are poor health and obesity. African-Americans suffer from diabetes twice as often as other Americans, and over half the African-American population is overweight. African-Americans also have a higher chance of suffering from strokes or cancer than any other ethnic group.

Regardless of your ethnicity, *Neo Soul* is meant to broaden your soul food experience. You can still experience the comforts of home-style soul food, but with a little more effort, you can find alternatives that are healthy for you. These recipes are meant to be made with organic ingredients. Organic foods are chemical- and hormone-free, use no preservatives, and offer great taste. In addition to the recipes, we've included tips for easy preparation.

I'm very proud of my soul food tradition. I want to give people the best food that I can by offering alternatives that will enable everyone to live a healthier lifestyle. If the most famous soul food restaurant in the country can make those changes, then you can too!

# • STRUCTURE HOUSE •

Structure House was extremely important to me in my journey to weight loss. It was founded in 1977 by Gerard J. Musante, a clinical psychologist who specialized in working with overweight patients. The staff includes experts in psychology, nutrition, and fitness. They emphasize nutrition, exercise, and stress management. I couldn't possibly say too many nice things about them, and I certainly wouldn't be where I am today if I hadn't gone to Structure House all those years ago. You can contact Structure House by telephone at 800-553-0052 or 919-493-0205, by e-mail at info@structurehouse.com, or by regular mail at the following address: Structure House, 3017 Pickett Road, Durham, NC 27705.

# 2

# Breakfast Foods
# and Breads

Breakfast always reminds me of my childhood summers in South Carolina, which I usually spent with my great-grandmother Julia Pressley. Her kitchen was always filled with the aroma of fresh coffee from a pot or two simmering on the stove. Breakfast was always an early meal, but not necessarily a short one.

Like many soul food meals, breakfast often consisted of many dishes and an assortment of sides. Grandma Julia was a big believer in grits. I never saw her cook a breakfast without some grits on the side. To this day, whenever I eat grits I think of my great-grandmother.

Breakfast is extremely important. You get to start your day with energy and a good meal. And if you skip breakfast, you're more likely to snack later in the day. I like to start my breakfast with a fruit bowl and yogurt. You can try different fruits and different yogurts for some variety. Personally, I look forward to watermelon season every summer—it's my all-time favorite fruit with yogurt. A small bowl, and I'm ready for anything . . . a morning run, a meeting in midtown, or tackling a brunch for a hundred people.

If you have a real sweet tooth, you can sprinkle a dash of Splenda—a sugar substitute that's actually made from sugar—over your fruit and yogurt.

## Uptown Biscuits

The secret to making great biscuits is to be sure that you do not work the butter in too much. The particles really should be pea-sized. This allows for the butter to create spaces during the baking process. The result? Flaky, moist biscuits. Also, be sure not to work the dough too much. Overkneading will result in a poor-quality biscuit. The less time there is between the bowl and the baking sheet, the better. The use of lowfat or soymilk helps make these biscuits a bit healthier than many others.
*Serves 12*

Nonstick cooking spray
2½ cups unbleached all-purpose flour
2½ tablespoons baking powder
1 teaspoon kosher salt
1¾ sticks butter, cut into small pieces
1¾ cups 1% milk or soymilk

1. Preheat the oven to 425 degrees. Spray a baking sheet with nonstick cooking spray and set it aside.

2. Place the flour, baking powder, and salt in a large bowl and mix. Add the butter pieces and begin to cut* the butter into the flour with one or two forks or a pastry cutter,† until the particles are the size of green peas.

3. Add the milk and stir until it is all completely combined.

4. Dust a clean counter surface with flour and turn the dough out onto the counter. Knead only minimally. The dough should be soft and supple.

5. Roll the dough out flat (about ⅛ inch thick) and cut 3-inch rounds with a biscuit cutter or small juice glass.

6. Place the biscuits on the baking sheet and bake for 12 to 15 minutes, until golden brown.

**NUTRITIONAL INFORMATION PER SERVING**

235 CALORIES  •  4G PROTEIN  •  14G FAT  •  175MG SODIUM

*"Cut": To mix solid fat into a dry ingredient until the combination mixture is in small particles.

†Pastry cutter: A half-moon-shaped implement consisting of 5 or 6 U-shaped sturdy wires, with both ends attached to a wooden handle. It is used to cut fat into flour because no heat is transferred to the wires from the hands during use. It's also faster than using a knife.

# Mixed Fruit and Yogurt Parfait

Dishes like this one are a big part of my plan to lose weight and keep it off. It takes virtually no effort to make, and it satisfies my breakfast cravings many mornings. There are quite a few healthy, nutritious ingredients, too.   *Serves 8*

1 pint raspberries, lightly rinsed

1 pint blueberries, lightly rinsed

1 pound seedless grapes, washed and cut in half

½ cantaloupe, peeled and cut into small chunks

½ honeydew, peeled and cut into small chunks

½ pineapple, peeled and cut into small chunks, or 8 ounces fresh
    pineapple chunks

1 pint strawberries, rinsed and cut in half

1 cup honey

1 quart plain yogurt

¾ cup granola

1. Reserving some berries for garnish, combine all the fruit in a large bowl and mix well. Set the fruit aside.
2. In a separate medium-sized bowl, combine the honey and yogurt. Set the mixture aside.
3. Set out 4 to 6 parfait-style glasses or wineglasses. Place a layer of fruit in the bottom of each glass. Next, place a layer of the yogurt mixture and then a layer of the granola. Continue layering until each glass is full, ending with the yogurt.

4. Garnish with berries. For example, a half strawberry, a raspberry, or three blueberries in the center.

Tɪᴘ: Sometimes food can be scary. Pineapple tastes great but it can be difficult to cut. As a solution, many major supermarkets now carry pineapple, honeydew, and cantaloupe cleaned and nicely cut, in the produce "grab and go" section.

### NUTRITIONAL INFORMATION PER SERVING
384 CALORIES • 8G PROTEIN • 7G FAT • 67MG SODIUM

## Oatmeal and Apples

One of the most important things I've taught myself to do over the last few years is to read food labels. I always choose foods that are low in saturated fat, total fat, cholesterol, and calories. The most important (and easiest) thing you can do today to eat healthier is begin using lowfat milk in recipes that call for milk.   *Serves 4*

4 cups water, 1% milk, or lowfat milk

1 pinch kosher salt

½ tablespoon butter

2 teaspoons brown sugar, firmly packed

4 apples, cored, peeled, and diced
   (use your favorite variety)

2 cups dry rolled oats

2 teaspoons cinnamon

1. In a large saucepan over high heat, bring the 4 cups of water or milk to a boil with the salt.
2. In a small skillet, melt the butter and sugar over medium heat. Add the apples to the skillet and cook for 3 to 5 minutes, until the apples are soft. Remove them from the heat.
3. Stir the oats into the boiling water. Stir for 10 to 15 minutes, to avoid lumps, until the mixture becomes thick and smooth.
4. Fold the apples into the oatmeal.
5. Divide into bowls and sprinkle each serving with cinnamon.

TIP: Do not hesitate to experiment with this by using your favorite fruit of another variety. Try bananas, strawberries, blueberries, or peaches. Always remember to go with what is in season.

## NUTRITIONAL INFORMATION PER SERVING

265 CALORIES · 11G PROTEIN · 6G FAT · 154MG SODIUM

# • HOW MUCH IS A "SERVING SIZE"? •

It might be smaller than you would like. For example, according to the USDA, 1 serving size equals ½ cup of mashed potatoes or cooked rice, 1 medium apple, and 1 slice of whole-grain bread. Remember: control your weight by controlling your portion sizes.

## Oatmeal Pancakes

I am a big advocate of preventing childhood obesity. I know how much I suffered growing up fat and picked on. If I can help even one kid eat right and slim down, it's all worth it. The number-one thing parents can do to keep their child from gaining too much weight is avoid prepared foods with extra sugar. Start your family's day off right with a light and healthy breakfast. *Serves 4*

2 cups oatmeal flour *
5 teaspoons baking powder

*Found in large grocery stores, and health food and organic shops.*

1 tablespoon cinnamon

1 teaspoon kosher salt

2 cups egg substitute

2 cups lowfat milk or soymilk

⅔ cup butter, melted and allowed to cool

3 tablespoons honey

1 teaspoon vanilla

2 tablespoons raisins

Nonstick cooking spray

1. Whisk together the flour, baking powder, cinnamon, and salt in a large bowl until completely combined.

2. In a medium-sized bowl, whisk together the egg substitute, milk, butter, honey, and vanilla until completely combined.

3. Fold the wet mixture into the dry mixture. When thoroughly combined, fold in the raisins.

4. Spray a large skillet or griddle pan with nonstick cooking spray. Place two heaping tablespoons of batter (one pancake) on the heated surface. Cook on one side until the edges firm up and bubbles start to form, about 3 to 5 minutes. Flip and cook on the other side for an additional 1 to 2 minutes.

VARIATION: You can also add 2 cups of whole oats with raisins in step 3 for dense pancakes.

NUTRITIONAL INFORMATION PER SERVING

529 CALORIES · 26G PROTEIN · 24G FAT · 821MG SODIUM

## Southern Omelet

~~~~~~~~~~~~~~~~~

Here's a tip for the next time you prepare an omelet: Use a rubber spatula to fold one half of the omelet over the other, like a book. This will give an authentic omelet-style presentation.  *Serves 4*

Nonstick cooking spray
½ red pepper, diced
½ small onion, diced
2 cups egg substitute
1 teaspoon hot sauce

1. Spray a medium skillet with nonstick cooking spray and cook the pepper and onion over medium heat until soft.
2. Add the egg substitute and cook until firm.
3. Garnish with hot sauce.

**NUTRITIONAL INFORMATION PER SERVING**

115 CALORIES · 15G PROTEIN · 5G FAT · 235MG SODIUM

## Pan-Fried Home Fries with Garlic

~~~~~~~~~~~~~~~~~

Fried potatoes go with so many dishes, and nearly everyone loves them! The hint of garlic in my recipe makes this potato dish delicious and memorable. Just have a small serving instead of a typically large portion and you can include this in your diet every so often.

The trick to cooking home fries is not to stir them or turn them until a nice crust is formed. *Serves 6*

1 pound potatoes, cut into medium dice
1 tablespoon butter
2 tablespoons olive oil
1 garlic clove, minced
1 onion, chopped
1 red pepper, chopped
1 green pepper, chopped
Kosher salt and fresh black pepper to taste

1. Place the potatoes in a large pot and cover them with water. Cook over medium heat for 10 to 12 minutes, until they begin to soften. Remove the potatoes from the heat and drain them.
2. In a large skillet over medium-high heat, melt the butter and then add the olive oil. When the mixture begins to sizzle, add the garlic, onion, and red and green peppers. Cook for 2 minutes and add the potatoes.
3. Lower the heat to medium and continue cooking for 8 to 10 minutes, turning once, until a crust begins to form on the bottom of the softened potatoes.

NUTRITIONAL INFORMATION PER SERVING
122 CALORIES · 3G PROTEIN · 13G FAT · 15MG SODIUM

## Spinach and Cheese Bake

A quintessential soul food favorite! Except this version has fewer calories than the ones I ate years ago.   *Serves 8*

1 pound skim-milk ricotta

1 pound skim-milk mozzarella

1-pound bag fresh spinach, blanched, shocked with cold water, and
   chopped

1 egg white

1 garlic clove, crushed

2 stalks fresh thyme, stripped (leaves only)  (see below)

## • HOW DO YOU STRIP AN HERB? •

Take a stalk of thyme, rosemary, or oregano between your thumb and forefinger and pull in a downward motion to remove the leaves. Some recipes may call for the leaves and not the stalks. You can always save the stalks though, and add them to soups, stocks, or sauces.

1 small onion, chopped

Nonstick cooking spray

1. Preheat the oven to 350 degrees.
2. In a large bowl, combine all ingredients except the cooking spray and mix well.
3. Coat a 9-inch pie plate with nonstick cooking spray and pour the mixture into the pie plate.
4. Bake for 45 to 50 minutes, or until set.

**NUTRITIONAL INFORMATION PER SERVING**

243 CALORIES · 23G PROTEIN · 14G FAT · 391MG SODIUM

## Mushroom and Spinach Omelet

Studies show that African-Americans generally accept larger body sizes and have less guilt about over-eating. This can lead to obesity and other health problems. For many years, that was the sad story of my life. But I turned it around with exercise and healthy eating, like the following omelet recipe, which includes excellent vegetables and some dairy products. *Serves 4*

1 tablespoon olive oil

1 medium onion, cut into small dice

4 ounces mushrooms, sliced (use your favorite variety)

1-pound bag baby spinach

Kosher salt and fresh black pepper to taste

2 cups egg whites

4 ounces goat cheese, crumbled

1. In a large skillet, preheat the oil over medium-high heat. Add the onion and mushrooms and cook for about 5 minutes, until they are soft.
2. Add the bag of spinach and season the vegetables with salt and pepper. With tongs, turn the onion, mushrooms, and spinach until the spinach is completely wilted.
3. Pour in the egg whites and cook for 3 to 5 minutes, until they begin to firm.
4. Sprinkle the goat cheese on top and fold the egg whites over. Continue to cook for 2 to 3 minutes.

**NUTRITIONAL INFORMATION PER SERVING**

296 CALORIES · 26G PROTEIN · 17G FAT · 389MG SODIUM

## Walnut Coffee Cake

Here's a cake recipe that works well as a breakfast treat. Remember to consume treats like this in moderation.   *Serves 12*

3 cups whole-wheat flour or all-purpose flour

2 teaspoons baking powder

1 teaspoon baking soda

1 teaspoon cinnamon

2 cups egg whites

1½ sticks butter, melted and allowed to cool

1 cup honey

2 cups lowfat milk or soymilk

1 cup chopped walnuts, toasted

Nonstick cooking spray

1. Preheat the oven to 350 degrees.
2. In a large bowl, sift together the flour, baking powder, baking soda, and cinnamon.
3. In another bowl combine the egg whites, butter, honey, and milk.
4. Fold the wet ingredients into the dry ingredients with a rubber spatula. Be sure to work and scrape from the sides as well as from the bottom. When the wet and dry ingredients are incorporated, fold in half the nuts.
5. Spray a coffee ring or like pan with nonstick cooking spray and pour the batter in. Sprinkle the remaining walnuts on top.
6. Bake for 35 to 45 minutes, until a toothpick inserted in the center of the cake comes out clean (see page 143).
7. Remove the cake from the oven and place on a cooling rack. When it is completely cool, cut and serve.

NUTRITIONAL INFORMATION PER SERVING

294 CALORIES · 8G PROTEIN · 18G FAT · 156MG SODIUM

# Banana Bread

~~~~~~~~~~~~

Seems to me my grandmother's kitchen always had something bubbling up on top of the stove . . . and something baking in the oven and sending sweet aromas through the house. Banana bread, zucchini bread, and others were part of our family's kitchen. Yours, too, probably. You'll see with this recipe, which contains a bit less butter and sugar, you don't have to give them up to enjoy a healthier diet.   *Serves 12*

Nonstick cooking spray
1 cup flour
¼ cup sugar
1 teaspoon baking powder
⅓ teaspoon baking soda
½ teaspoon kosher salt
¼ cup chopped walnuts
3 eggs
1 cup puréed bananas
½ stick butter, melted and allowed to cool

1. Preheat the oven to 375 degrees.
2. Spray nonstick cooking spray in a standard size (9-inch) loaf pan.
3. In a large bowl, whisk together the flour, sugar, baking powder, baking soda, salt, and nuts.
4. In a smaller bowl, whisk together the eggs, bananas, and butter. Fold slowly into the dry ingredients.

5. Pour the entire batter into the pan and bake for about 50 minutes, or until a toothpick inserted in the center comes out clean (see page 143).

6. Remove from pan and let cool on a wire rack.

**NUTRITIONAL INFORMATION PER SERVING:**

139 CALORIES · 4G PROTEIN · 7G FAT · 138MG SODIUM

# Zucchini Bread

In South Carolina my family often grew their own squash and would use some of it for this excellent bread. It's delicious and a healthy treat.

*Serves 16*

Nonstick cooking spray

1 cup white sugar

¼ cup brown sugar, firmly packed

¾ cup vegetable oil

2 eggs

2 cups flour

2½ teaspoons cinnamon

¾ teaspoon baking powder

¾ teaspoon baking soda

½ teaspoon salt

1½ cups finely chopped zucchini

½ cup chopped walnuts

1. Preheat the oven to 350 degrees. Spray two standard (9-inch) loaf pans with nonstick cooking spray.
2. In a large bowl, combine the white sugar, brown sugar, oil, and eggs. Mix well.
3. In another bowl, mix the flour, cinnamon, baking powder, baking soda, and salt. Add to the egg mixture and blend.
4. Carefully fold in the zucchini and nuts. Divide the mixture into the two greased loaf pans and bake for 55 minutes.

**NUTRITIONAL INFORMATION PER SERVING**

281 CALORIES • 4G PROTEIN • 24G FAT • 118MG SODIUM

## Southern Cornbread

Cornbread is a classic Southern soul food. And here is a good place to talk about one of the most important classic African-American chefs, Mrs. Abby Fisher. More than a hundred years ago, Mrs. Fisher lived in California and made her living as a cook and caterer. She was, as far as we know, the first black American woman to write down her own recipes. Her cookbook, which included 160 recipes, was first published in 1881. *Serves 8*

2¼ cups 1% milk or soymilk
¼ stick butter
1 tablespoon honey
1 teaspoon kosher salt

⅔ cup yellow cornmeal

Nonstick cooking spray

3 egg yolks, well beaten

3 egg whites, beaten to stiff peaks

1. Preheat the oven to 375 degrees.
2. Heat the milk in a large saucepan over high heat until near scalding. Add the butter, honey, and salt. Slowly stir in the cornmeal. Cook for 1 minute. Remove the pan from the heat and let cool a few minutes.
3. Spray a 4-cup casserole dish with nonstick cooking spray and set aside.
4. Stir the cornmeal mixture into the egg yolks. Then fold in the egg whites.
5. Pour the batter into the prepared baking dish and bake for 35 to 40 minutes, until the top is golden brown.

VARIATION: To make hush puppies, during step 3, fold in ½ cup sliced scallions and ½ teaspoon cayenne pepper. Eliminate step 5. Instead, deep-fry heaping tablespoonfuls of the batter for down-home hush puppies.

NUTRITIONAL INFORMATION PER SERVING

130 CALORIES · 6G PROTEIN · 6G FAT · 57MG SODIUM

# 3

# Salads and Soups

A soup and a salad can be a light yet satisfying meal, but sometimes it's not as simple as it sounds. When you're trying to lose weight, everybody tells you to eat a salad. So I did. Only I loaded my salads with so much dressing, so much cheese, and so much meat that I never lost any weight. If you're eating a salad, make sure it's a real salad.

The other problem with traditional soul food is that the "salads" aren't really salads at all, like potato salad and macaroni salad. Now I try to eat healthier salads, like a three-bean salad, or a light chicken salad. Just remember to try to put as many greens as you can in your bowl before you add meat or cheese.

The same thing goes for soup. If you're mopping up your soup with huge chunks of cornbread—as I've seen people do in the restaurant— then you're not really eating a light meal. Soups can be hearty and refreshing without lots of fat. One thing to remember: No matter what soup you like, try to make sure it's low in sodium. Many soups can be high in salt, which adds to water weight and is especially bad for those with high blood pressure. It's easy to make a tasty soup without overdoing the salt—just add some spice instead.

## Alison's Summer Salad

Salads don't have to be side dishes. If you have the right combination of nutritious ingredients, a salad becomes a meal. Just ask my friend Alison, who shared this recipe with me a few years ago.   *Serves 8*

⅓ cup red wine vinegar

⅓ cup balsamic vinegar

¾ cup extra-virgin olive oil

1½ teaspoons dried oregano, crushed

5 very ripe tomatoes, cut into quarters

2 pounds string beans, washed, with ends trimmed

1 large can hearts of palm, drained and cut into quarters

¼ cup lowfat Parmesan

In a large bowl, combine the two vinegars, oil, and crushed oregano. Whisk well. Add the tomatoes, string beans, and hearts of palm. Mix until well combined. Chill for at least an hour. Sprinkle with the cheese before serving.

**NUTRITIONAL INFORMATION PER SERVING**

242 CALORIES · 4G PROTEIN · 20G FAT · 98MG SODIUM

# Avocado Pasta Salad

Avocado is one of the fruits highest in fat. But according to several studies, avocado can help reduce cholesterol. *Serves 6*

1 pound pasta of your choice

¼ cup plus 1 cup olive oil

5 avocados

½ bunch parsley, chopped

½ bunch cilantro, chopped

2 tablespoons lime juice

½ jalapeño pepper, minced

2 garlic cloves, minced

½ teaspoon kosher salt

4 plum tomatoes, seeded and diced

1 red onion, cut into small dice

1. Cook the pasta according to the package directions. Remove the cooked pasta from the heat and drain while running under cold water for 5 to 8 minutes. Toss the pasta with ¼ oil to prevent sticking. Place the pasta in a bowl and chill.

2. Peel and cut one avocado in half lengthwise and remove the pit.

3. To make the dressing, combine the halved avocado, half the parsley, half the cilantro, and the lime juice, jalapeño, garlic, and salt in a food processor or strong blender. Blend until all ingredients are well combined. Add the 1 cup oil in a stream, blending until the mixture is creamy. The dressing should resemble mayonnaise in consistency. If it

begins to get too thick, add some water to loosen it up. Add only a small amount of oil (¼ cup or so) at a time. Set aside.

4. Peel 4 of the avocados, halve them, remove the pits, and dice. In a large bowl, combine the chilled pasta, diced avocados, tomatoes, onion, and remaining parsley and cilantro. Mix until well combined.

5. Fold in the avocado dressing. The salad should hold together.

VARIATION: Add grilled chicken—after the dressing is added or as a side dish—for a complete meal.

NUTRITIONAL INFORMATION PER SERVING

313 CALORIES • 12G PROTEIN • 7G FAT • 149MG SODIUM

## • BALSAMIC REDUCTION •

Sometimes the balsamic vinegar you buy in your local supermarket is a little thin. To give it more depth, pour it into a medium-sized stainless-steel pot. Simmer over low heat until the vinegar resembles syrup in its consistency. Remove from the heat and immediately chill in an ice bath. Store in your refrigerator. This vinegar will make a richer salad dressing as well as a nice topping for fresh tomatoes.

# Broccoli and Corn Salad

The benefits of broccoli are amazing. It's high in fiber and beta-carotene, a powerful antioxidant that your body will convert into vitamin A.
*Serves 8*

3 cups broccoli, florets only

2 cups fresh corn

1 red pepper, cut into small dice

1 yellow pepper, cut into small dice

2 celery stalks, cut into small dice

1 red onion, cut into small dice

2 cups Balsamic Reduction (see page 44)

1 cup extra-virgin olive oil

In a large bowl, toss all the ingredients together until well combined. Chill for 20 minutes and serve.

### NUTRITIONAL INFORMATION PER SERVING

316 CALORIES · 3G PROTEIN · 28G FAT · 65MG SODIUM

# Cajun Jumbo Shrimp Salad

~~~~~~~~~~~~~~~~~~~~~~~~~~~~~~~~

There are so many health benefits associated with eating seafood on a regular basis. Not only is it an excellent protein food, certain types of seafood are a good source of omega-3 fatty acids, which may help prevent heart disease and certain types of cancers. Shrimp is one of my favorite types of seafood, and this recipe really satisfies.  *Serves 4*

2 tablespoons Cajun seasoning
6 tablespoons olive oil
1 pound jumbo shrimp, peeled and deveined
3 heads green leaf lettuce, washed and chopped
2 pints (4 cups) yellow pear tomatoes, halved
6 scallions, sliced
½ bunch cilantro, washed and chopped fine

1. In a plastic bag, combine the Cajun seasoning and 2 tablespoons of the olive oil. Knot the end and shake vigorously. Open the bag and add the shrimp. Shake again until all the pieces are well coated. Set aside the bag with the shrimp inside.
2. Add 2 tablespoons of the oil to a large skillet and place over high heat. When the skillet begins to smoke, add the shrimp and cook. Slide the skillet back and forth gently over the heat to cook the shrimp on all sides. Look for the shrimp to turn pink and curl as a sign they are done. This will take 6 to 8 minutes.
3. When the shrimp are fully cooked, remove from the heat, saving the drippings from the skillet, and chill immediately for at least 30 minutes.

4. Combine the lettuce, tomatoes, scallions, and cilantro in a large bowl. Add the chilled shrimp, pan drippings, and remaining 2 tablespoons oil. Toss until well combined. Chill until ready to serve.

NUTRITIONAL INFORMATION PER SERVING

393 CALORIES · 30G PROTEIN · 23G FAT · 270MG SODIUM

## Carrot and Raisin Salad

Carrot lovers proclaim that this little orange vegetable can help slow aging, treat asthma and high blood pressure, and lessen skin wrinkles. I don't know about all of that, but carrots remain one of my favorite salad and snack foods.   *Serves 4*

½ cup lowfat mayonnaise
2 tablespoons honey
½ teaspoon kosher salt
1 pound carrots, peeled and shredded
½ cup raisins

In a large bowl, combine the mayonnaise, honey, and salt. Mix well. Add the carrots and raisins and mix until well coated.

NUTRITIONAL INFORMATION PER SERVING

185 CALORIES · 2G PROTEIN · 4G FAT · 540MG SODIUM

# Chef's Salad

In 1980, 5 percent of the teenage population was obese. Today, nearly 20 percent is. Families can help their young adults eat right and feel better about themselves by providing the right foods. Most teens love chef salads. Here is my favorite version, and it's one I think will please even your teenager. *Serves 8*

16 large romaine lettuce leaves
1 pound turkey breast, cut into medium dice
1 pound grilled chicken, sliced thin
8 hard-boiled eggs, sliced
1 red onion, sliced thin
2 yellow peppers, sliced thin
2 pints (4 cups) pear tomatoes, halved
2 cups lowfat cheddar cheese
1 cucumber, deseeded* and sliced
Your favorite dressing

*"Deseeded": to deseed a cucumber, peel it and cut it in half lengthwise. Using a teaspoon or tablespoon, scrape down the center where the seeds are and discard them. This will keep excess water out of your salads.*

For each individual salad, start with four large lettuce leaves as a base. With a salad plate in front of you, arrange one-quarter of the turkey at 6 o'clock and one-quarter of the chicken at 12 o'clock. Next, place one-quarter of the egg slices at 3 o'clock and one-quarter of the onion slices at 9 o'clock. The peppers go between nine and twelve, and the tomatoes are placed between twelve and three; the cheese goes between three and six; finally, place the cucumber between six and nine. Drizzle with your favorite dressing and serve.

NUTRITIONAL INFORMATION PER SERVING

423 CALORIES  •  52G PROTEIN  •  17G FAT  •  349MG SODIUM

## Thousand Island Dressing

The trick to hearty, healthy salads is twofold: Use the freshest ingredients you can find and never drown the salad in dressing. The best dressings are fragrant and delicious, but you want just enough on your salad to hint of taste and flavor. *Serves 12*

1 cup chopped sweet gherkins

1 cup lowfat mayonnaise

¼ cup tomato sauce

2 tablespoons honey

2 teaspoons garlic powder

1 teaspoon kosher salt

1 teaspoon fresh black pepper

Combine all the ingredients in a large bowl, stir vigorously, and chill for 1 hour.

NUTRITIONAL INFORMATION PER SERVING

57 CALORIES  •  .1G PROTEIN  •  3G FAT  •  431MG SODIUM

# Chopped Garden Salad

~~~~~~~~~~~~~~~~~~~~~~~~~

The secret to this great salad is watercress. Watercress is one of the foods highest in lysine, an amino acid the body needs for growth and to repair tissue damage. You need to get it from outside sources like watercress because the body doesn't produce its own.   *Serves 4*

2 heads romaine lettuce, shredded

2 carrots, peeled and shredded

1 bunch watercress, washed, stems removed, and leaves chopped

2 cups Brussels sprouts, cleaned and shredded

2 celery stalks, washed and finely chopped

1-pound bag baby spinach, chopped

3 cups broccoli florets, washed and chopped

Dressing (optional)

In a large bowl, mix all the ingredients together. Add a small amount of dressing, if you so choose, and chill for 10 to 15 minutes.

### NUTRITIONAL INFORMATION PER SERVING

134 CALORIES • 29G PROTEIN • 56G FAT • 189MG SODIUM

# Balsamic Vinaigrette

Several of my recipes call for balsamic vinegar. It's aged vinegar that was originally made in Modena, Italy, and it typically costs more than regular vinegar. You should add balsamic vinegar to your kitchen. It's unique, fragrant, and delicious. *Serves 10*

2 shallots, finely chopped

1 teaspoon fresh thyme leaves

1 teaspoon honey

¼ cup Balsamic Reduction (see page 44)

1 tablespoon Dijon mustard

1 cup olive oil

Salt and fresh black pepper to taste

In a blender, combine all the ingredients except the oil, salt, and pepper. With the blender on, slowly add the oil. When the mixture begins to thicken, turn the blender off. Season the vinaigrette to taste with salt and pepper.

**NUTRITIONAL INFORMATION PER SERVING**

126 CALORIES • 1G PROTEIN • 13G FAT • 11MG SODIUM

# Elena's Asparagus Salad

Asparagus is a member of the lily family (as are garlic, onions, and leeks), and it's filled with nutrients. It's an excellent source of folic acid, a significant source of vitamin C, and a good source of vitamin A.

This salad is best if it is chilled overnight, to allow the vegetables to absorb the balsamic vinegar.   *Serves 4*

Pinch of kosher salt
1 pound green asparagus, cleaned, with tough ends trimmed
8 pieces pickled okra, drained and cut into small rounds
1 small onion, sliced thin
½ cup Balsamic Reduction (see page 44)
Fresh black pepper to taste
½ cup crumbled blue cheese

1. Fill a large pot with water three-quarters of the way. Add a pinch of salt and place over high heat.
2. Prepare an ice bath for the cooked asparagus.
3. When the water boils, place the asparagus in the pot for 3 to 5 minutes only. This will partially cook it. The asparagus should be bright green and just beginning to bend when removed from the boiling water. Immediately shock the asparagus by placing it in the ice bath until cool. Remove from the ice water, drain, and pat dry.
4. Cut the asparagus into pieces that are 2 inches long and place the pieces in a large bowl. Add the okra, onion, and balsamic reduction. Toss. Season with black pepper to taste.

5. Add the blue cheese to the top, cover, and chill at least 4 hours before serving.

# Heirloom Tomato Salad

An heirloom tomato is any tomato from a variety grown from seeds that were used before the arrival of mega-agriculture. Heirlooms are available at farmers' markets, roadside stands, and specialty grocers, and maybe in your own backyard.  *Serves 4*

5 large heirloom tomatoes, thickly sliced
1 red onion, thinly sliced
Salt and fresh black pepper to taste
Leaves of 4 stalks fresh oregano
¼ cup extra-virgin olive oil
2 tablespoons Balsamic Reduction (page 44)
½ cup crumbled blue cheese

On a plate, arrange rows of tomato, onion, tomato, onion, and so on, with a slight overlap. They should resemble shingles on a roof. Sprinkle with salt, pepper, and oregano leaves. Drizzle the oil and balsamic reduction on top. Cover the plate with plastic wrap and chill for at least 1 hour before serving. Sprinkle the crumbled blue cheese on top of the salad immediately before serving.

NUTRITIONAL INFORMATION PER SERVING

197 CALORIES · 7G PROTEIN · 12G FAT · 262MG SODIUM

## Black-Eyed Pea Salad

There's nothing that captures the "soul" of soul food more than black-eyed peas. I consider it the African-American signature dish. Black-eyed peas were a seasonal vegetable in the South, but now you can have them anytime at all.    *Serves 6*

3 cups prepared or canned black-eyed peas, rinsed and drained

1 green pepper, cut into small dice

2 red peppers, cut into small dice

6 celery stalks, chopped

1 onion, chopped

¼ cup honey

2 cups cider vinegar

1 garlic clove, minced

2 teaspoons kosher salt

2 teaspoons fresh black pepper

1 cup extra-virgin olive oil

Toss all the ingredients in a large bowl until completely combined. Chill at least 30 minutes before serving.

**NUTRITIONAL INFORMATION PER SERVING**

494 CALORIES  •  7G PROTEIN  •  36G FAT  •  396MG SODIUM

## Lindsey's Pasta Salad

I always thought one of the marks of a good picnic was a high-quality pasta salad. It seems to be a staple of any outdoor summer outing, whether in the Hamptons, New York, or Hemingway, South Carolina. This is my own healthy version.  *Serves 8*

1 pound pasta

1 cup lowfat mayonnaise

½ red pepper, chopped

½ green pepper, chopped

4 celery stalks, chopped

1 small onion, chopped

Salt and fresh black pepper, to taste

1. Cook the pasta according to the package directions. Drain and let cool. Set aside.

2. In a large bowl, combine the mayonnaise, red pepper, green pepper,

celery, and onion. Mix well. Add the cooled pasta. Using a rubber spat-ula, fold the dressing in until the pasta is all well coated.

TIP: Pasta will absorb a great deal of dressing. If you've prepared the salad well ahead of time, be sure to add more dressing right before serv-ing, in order to keep the salad moist and delicious.

NUTRITIONAL INFORMATION PER SERVING

173 CALORIES · 7G PROTEIN · 1G FAT · 40MG SODIUM

# Mom's Healthy Garden Salad and Fresh Vinaigrette

My mother, Bedelia, is just as concerned with healthy eating as I am, and she has even convinced my grandmother to make changes in Sylvia's Restaurant. Here's a salad with a great low-calorie dressing that Mom eats nearly every day of the week. She drizzles on some of the vinaigrette dressing (see page 51) to make a perfect light lunch.    *Serves 4*

VINAIGRETTE

1 shallot, minced

1 tablespoon grated Parmesan cheese

1 tablespoon Balsamic Reduction (see page 44)

3 tablespoons olive oil

SALAD

2 cups organic spinach

2 cups baby arugula

½ head red leaf lettuce, washed and chopped

1 cucumber, peeled, deseeded,* and sliced

1 pint (2 cups) grape tomatoes, halved

1 yellow pepper, sliced

½ head fennel, thinly sliced

1 red onion, thinly sliced

Salt and fresh black pepper to taste

1. To make the dressing, combine the shallot, cheese, and balsamic reduction in a small bowl. Whisk in the oil and set aside.
2. To make the salad, combine the spinach, arugula, lettuce, cucumber, tomatoes, yellow pepper, fennel, and red onion in a large bowl. Pour the vinaigrette in at the side of the bowl and toss the salad from the bottom until completely coated.
3. Season with salt and pepper to taste.

*"Deseeded": To deseed a cucumber, peel it and cut it in half lengthwise. Using a teaspoon or tablespoon, scrape down the center where the seeds are and discard them. This will keep excess water out of your salads.

TIP: Thinly sliced fennel gives summer salads an unusual, refreshing flavor that is a great complement to many dishes.

**NUTRITIONAL INFORMATION PER SERVING**

65 CALORIES · 5G PROTEIN · 1G FAT · 59MG SODIUM

# Pan-Fried Catfish Salad

Be sure to use reduced-fat and low-calorie salad dressings. If you don't like those, try vinaigrette. I've included a couple of terrific dressing recipes in *Neo Soul*. The following catfish salad recipe, however, calls for a simple lemon juice and oil dressing. You can experiment with a dressing of your own, too. (But never drown a salad with it!)   *Serves 6*

¼ cup cornmeal

2 tablespoons cornstarch

1 tablespoon Mrs. Dash seasoning blend

2 teaspoons kosher salt

2 teaspoons fresh black pepper

1 pound catfish, fried

2 tablespoons plus ½ cup olive oil

2 heads romaine lettuce, chopped

1 cucumber, deseeded (see page 48) and sliced

1 pint (2 cups) grape tomatoes, halved

Juice of 1 lemon

1. In a medium-sized bowl, combine the cornmeal, cornstarch, Mrs. Dash, salt, and pepper. Stir until all the ingredients are mixed thoroughly. Add the fish, a few pieces at a time, and coat with mixture.

2. Place a medium-sized skillet over high heat and add the 2 tablespoons oil. Add the fish and cook in batches for 8 to 10 minutes each, until cooked completely through. Place the fish on a paper towel–lined plate to allow it to cool and drain. Set aside.

3. In a large bowl, combine the lettuce, cucumber, and tomatoes. Add the fish pieces.

4. Drizzle the lemon juice and ½ cup oil over the entire salad and toss until well combined. Season with salt and pepper to taste.

**NUTRITIONAL INFORMATION PER SERVING**

259 CALORIES • 17G PROTEIN • 15G FAT • 369MG SODIUM

## Roasted Sweet Potato Salad

This is a great alternative to traditional potato salad because of the health benefits of sweet potatoes. You will notice that many of my recipes call for olive oil. That's because it is much healthier than other oils. To go even healthier, try using a nonstick cooking spray as a substitute as often as possible when a recipe calls for oil or butter. *Serves 4*

2 tablespoons olive oil

1 teaspoon fresh thyme leaves

1 teaspoon finely chopped fresh basil

2 teaspoons kosher salt

2 teaspoons fresh black pepper

2 sweet potatoes, cut into medium dice

¼ cup honey

2 tablespoons Dijon mustard

¾ cup lowfat mayonnaise

1. Preheat the oven to 350 degrees.

2. In a large bowl, combine the oil, thyme, and basil, 1 teaspoon of the salt, and 1 teaspoon of the pepper. Add the sweet potatoes and toss until well coated. Place the potatoes on a baking sheet and bake for 20 to 30 minutes, or until soft. Remove from the oven and let cool completely.

3. In a separate large bowl, whisk together the honey, mustard, and mayonnaise and the remaining salt and pepper. Whisk until well combined. Add the cooled potatoes and toss until well coated. Chill for at least 2 hours before serving.

TIP: Basil is a delicate herb, so be sure to use a very sharp knife when chopping. A dull knife will bruise the leaves and cause them to turn black.

NUTRITIONAL INFORMATION PER SERVING

322 CALORIES · 2G PROTEIN · 8G FAT · 996MG SODIUM

# Shaved Fennel, Grapefruit, and Avocado Salad

Check out the variety of fresh produce here! You will have your recommended daily amount of fruit just by enjoying this salad. *Serves 8*

3 large heads of fennel, sliced thin
2 pink grapefruits, sections only (no membranes)

2 avocados, peeled, pitted, and sliced

2 teaspoons kosher salt

2 teaspoons fresh black pepper

1 cup extra-virgin olive oil

2 cups fresh pink grapefruit juice

In a large bowl, combine the fennel, grapefruit sections, avocado, salt, and pepper. Toss gently. Add the oil and grapefruit juice and toss again until well combined. Chill for at least a couple of hours before serving.

**NUTRITIONAL INFORMATION PER SERVING**

411 CALORIES • 3G PROTEIN • 36G FAT • 52MG SODIUM

## Southwestern Chicken Salad

Did you know that garlic was once used to treat wounds and is considered a powerful healing herb? Here I use it along with other spices to add a real kick to chicken salad.    *Serves 6*

1 teaspoon cayenne pepper

1 teaspoon paprika

1 teaspoon garlic powder

1 teaspoon celery seeds or fennel seeds

1 teaspoon dry mustard powder or ground mustard seeds

1 teaspoon fresh black pepper

1 teaspoon kosher salt

½ teaspoon ground cumin

4 tablespoons olive oil

4 whole skinless chicken breasts

3 heads romaine lettuce, chopped

2 pints (4 cups) cherry tomatoes, halved

½ jalapeño pepper, minced

8 ounces pepperjack cheese, shredded

1. Preheat the oven to 350 degrees.
2. In a large bowl, combine the cayenne, paprika, garlic powder, celery seeds, dry mustard, pepper, salt, and cumin, and 2 tablespoons of the olive oil. Whisk together.
3. Add the chicken and thoroughly coat each piece. Place in a baking dish.
4. Bake the chicken for 20 minutes, or until cooked through. Remove from the oven and chill. With a rubber spatula, scrape any drippings from the baking dish and save in a small container (like a coffee cup).
5. When the chicken is cool, cut it into medium dice.
6. In another large bowl, combine the lettuce, tomatoes, jalapeño pepper, cheese, and diced chicken. Toss. Add the reserved pan drippings and the remaining 2 tablespoons oil and toss again until completely coated. Season with salt to taste.

NUTRITIONAL INFORMATION PER SERVING

379 CALORIES · 32G PROTEIN · 26G FAT · 651MG SODIUM

# Summer Corn Salad

~~~~~~~~~~~~~~~~~~~~~~

During my summers in South Carolina there were few treats I enjoyed more than eating fresh corn on the cob. This recipe tastes great with fresh corn, but you can make it with frozen or canned corn, too.
*Serves 4*

1 teaspoon honey

½ teaspoon kosher salt

½ teaspoon fresh black pepper

Juice of ½ lemon

1 tablespoon Balsamic Reduction (page 44)

⅓ cup olive oil

2 cups fresh corn kernels

1 small red onion, chopped

½ red pepper, cut into small dice

¼ cup finely chopped fresh parsley

1 garlic clove, minced

In a large bowl, combine the honey, salt, black pepper, lemon juice, and balsamic reduction. Whisk in the oil. Add the corn, onion, red pepper, parsley, and garlic. Toss until well blended. Chill for 1 hour before serving.

**NUTRITIONAL INFORMATION PER SERVING**

261 CALORIES • 3G PROTEIN • 19G FAT • 250MG SODIUM

# Three Bean Salad
# with Citrus Vinaigrette

~~~~~~~~~~~~~~~~~~

This is one of several dishes in *Neo Soul* that are perfect for vegetarians. It is loaded with natural vegan foods like fruit juices, vegetables, and beans. For best results, let it chill overnight so the beans can soak up the dressing.

*Serves 6*

½ cup fresh orange juice

½ cup fresh grapefruit juice

½ cup fresh lemon juice

½ cup fresh lime juice

2 tablespoons honey

2½ cups olive oil

Salt and fresh black pepper to taste (optional)

1 cup cooked pinto beans, drained and allowed to cool (or rinsed if canned)

1 cup cooked lima beans, drained and allowed to cool (or rinsed if canned)

1 cup cooked kidney beans, drained and allowed to cool (or rinsed if canned)

1 red onion, thinly sliced

½ bunch fresh parsley leaves, finely chopped

1. In a medium saucepan over high heat, combine the orange juice, grapefruit juice, lemon juice, lime juice, and honey. Boil until the liquid is reduced by half.

2. Remove the pan from the heat and let cool slightly. Begin to add the oil, slowly, in a stream, while whisking the juice reduction. First add 1 cup, then taste. If the juice is still too strong, continue to add ½ cup oil at a time, until you reach your desired flavor. You can season with salt and pepper, if you so choose. Set the pan aside.

3. In a large bowl, combine the beans, red onion, and parsley. Add the dressing and toss until the beans are completely coated.

4. Chill the salad for at least 2 hours before serving.

TIP: You may want to reserve some of the dressing so that you can toss the salad again right before serving.

### NUTRITIONAL INFORMATION PER SERVING
495 CALORIES · 6G PROTEIN · 72G FAT · 5OMG SODIUM

## B.J.'s Potato Salad

Every family has its own special (and sometimes *secret*) potato salad recipe. Here's superb potato salad from one of New York City's most in-demand chefs (she also happens to be a great friend of mine).    *Serves 8*

½ cup lowfat mayonnaise

¼ cup Dijon mustard

4 hard-boiled egg yolks, mashed

2 teaspoons white vinegar

1 cup of celery, washed and chopped

1 large onion, chopped

3 tablespoons parsley leaves, washed and chopped

Salt and fresh black pepper to taste

12 large Idaho potatoes, washed and cubed with skin on

1 tablespoon kosher salt

1. In a medium bowl, combine the mayonnaise, mustard, egg yolks, and vinegar. Whisk until smooth.
2. Fold in the celery and onion and half the parsley. Season with salt and pepper. Chill the dressing for about an hour.
3. Place the potatoes in a large pot with enough water to cover. Add the

# • LINDSEY'S TOP HEALTHY FOOD SUBSTITUTIONS •

1. Organic free-range chicken for ordinary chicken
2. Soy/vegetarian "meat" for real meat
3. Vegetable gravy (available in health food stores) rather than traditional gravy
4. Whole-wheat flour instead of white flour
5. Splenda instead of white sugar
6. For frying, grapeseed or olive oil
7. For baking, egg substitutes rather than whole eggs
8. Organic skim milk instead of whole milk

kosher salt to the water. Cook over medium heat until the potatoes are soft—but not mushy! Drain the potatoes and transfer them to a large mixing bowl.

4. Begin to slowly pour dressing over the *hot* potatoes. With a rubber spatula, fold constantly until the potatoes are covered, but reserve about one-third of the dressing for later use. Chill the salad for a minimum of 4 hours.

5. Before serving, adjust the salad with the remaining dressing and add additional salt and pepper if needed.

**NUTRITIONAL INFORMATION PER SERVING**

434 CALORIES  •  10G PROTEIN  •  13G FAT  •  786MG SODIUM

# Cole Slaw

Picnics, family gatherings, luncheons, winter, summer, year-round—this cole slaw recipe always pleases. To lower the sugar content even more, cut out the honey.   *Serves 6*

1 medium green cabbage, shredded
4 carrots, peeled and shredded using the large holes on a box
   grater
2 cups regular or lowfat mayonnaise
¼ cup honey
1 tablespoon cider vinegar

1 teaspoon fennel seeds or celery seeds, slightly crushed
Kosher salt and fresh black pepper to taste

1. Place the cabbage and carrots in a large mixing bowl and set aside.
2. To make the dressing, combine the mayonnaise, honey, vinegar, and fennel seeds in a medium mixing bowl. Stir and blend completely.
3. Begin adding the dressing to the cabbage mixture, ½ cup at a time, until all the vegetables are coated. Season with salt and pepper to taste and save any unused dressing.
4. Chill for at least 2 hours. Adjust the flavor with reserved dressing if needed before serving.

**NUTRITIONAL INFORMATION PER SERVING**

228 CALORIES · 2G PROTEIN · 11G FAT · 730MG SODIUM

## Easy Vegetable Stock

One way to add flavor to compensate for missing fat and salt in your food is to make your stock very rich by simmering it until half the liquid evaporates.

*Serves 8*

2 tablespoons olive oil
4 carrots, peeled and cut into large dice
2 large onions, peeled and quartered
2 heads of celery, cut into large dice

5 quarts water

1 medium cheese rind (see below)

1 bunch parsley stems, washed

1. In a large stockpot, heat the oil over medium-high heat.
2. Add the carrots, onions, and celery and stir for 6 to 8 minutes, until they are coated with oil and begin to brown.
3. Add the water, cheese rind, and parsley stems. Bring to a boil. Reduce the heat and simmer 45 minutes to 1 hour.

**NUTRITIONAL INFORMATION PER SERVING**

92 CALORIES  ·  2G PROTEIN  ·  3G FAT  ·  10MG SODIUM

Tip: Stock is a great way to add flavor whenever you cook. You can also adjust its flavor depending on what you add. For example, for sweeter stock add more carrot and less onion. For more of a salty taste, add a bigger piece of cheese rind. You can also use whatever vegetable scraps you have around. Cleaning mushrooms? Save the stems and add them to your stock. Asparagus ends or broccoli stems? Add them too. Make it your own by changing the combination.

## Chicken Vegetable Soup

Cheese rinds are a great way to add depth of flavor to soups and stocks without adding significant fat, calories, or carbohydrates. Ask your local market to save the rind for you or save your own rather than discarding it after the cheese has been used.   *Serves 8*

2 tablespoons olive oil

1 large onion, cut into small dice

1 garlic clove, minced

1 cup small dice celery

2 carrots, peeled and cut into small dice

1 whole chicken, cut into bite-sized pieces

3 quarts water

1 bunch parsley stems, washed and left whole

2 teaspoons kosher salt

2 teaspoons black peppercorns

1 small Parmesan rind

1. Heat the oil in a large soup pot, then add the onion and garlic and cook until soft. Add the celery and carrots and stir. Add the chicken and stir until it is coated with oil. Add the water, parsley stems, salt, peppercorns, and Parmesan rind and bring it all to a boil.
2. Reduce to a simmer and cook for 45 minutes to 1 hour, until the chicken is cooked through.
3. Be sure to remove the stems and rind before serving.

### NUTRITIONAL INFORMATION PER SERVING

354 CALORIES • 46G PROTEIN • 35G FAT • 650MG SODIUM

TIP: Parsley stems impart a unique flavor to all sorts of dishes without the chore of chopping parsley.

# Oxtail Soup

~~~~~~~~~~

Visit Sylvia's on Tuesdays and Wednesdays and you can order our famous oxtail soup. Here's my recipe for oxtail soup that captures all of the unique flavor with some healthier ingredients.   *Serves 4*

2 tablespoons olive oil

4 celery stalks, cut into medium dice

2 carrots, peeled and cut into small dice

2 onions, cut into small dice

½ teaspoon white vinegar

1 tablespoon Mrs. Dash seasoning blend

2 teaspoons kosher salt

2 teaspoons fresh black pepper

2½ quarts beef stock

1 pound oxtail (found at butcher shops and some grocers)

1. Coat the bottom of a large pot with the oil and place it over medium heat. Add the celery, carrots, and onions and cook until the vegetables are soft.
2. Add the vinegar, Mrs. Dash, salt, and pepper. Cook until the vinegar evaporates.
3. Add the stock and oxtail. Simmer for 1½ hours, until the meat is soft and falling off the bone. Skim the top layer of the soup as needed.

**NUTRITIONAL INFORMATION PER SERVING**

117 CALORIES · 3G PROTEIN · 11G FAT · 541MG SODIUM

# Yellow Split Pea Soup

~~~~~~~~~~~~~~~~~~~~~~~~~

Is there anything better on a cold winter evening than pea soup? If there is, I don't know about it.   *Serves 8*

2 tablespoons olive oil

1 large onion, cut into large dice

1 bunch scallions, sliced

1 sweet potato, cut into medium dice

1 white potato, cut into medium dice

1 celery stalk, cut into large dice

2 carrots, peeled and cut into medium dice

1 green banana, peeled and cut into medium rounds

2 cups fresh pumpkin, peeled, seeded, and cut into small cubes

½ cup coconut cream

2 teaspoons kosher salt

2 teaspoons fresh black pepper

1 tablespoon dried thyme

1 pound dried yellow peas, soaked and drained

2 quarts Easy Vegetable Stock (page 68)

1. Heat the oil in a large soup pot over a high heat. Add the onion and scallions and cook until soft.
2. Stir in the sweet potato, white potato, celery, carrots, banana, and pumpkin. Cook for 5 minutes to combine all the flavors.
3. Add the coconut cream, salt, pepper, and thyme. Stir to combine.
4. Add the peas and stock. Bring to a boil, lower the heat, and simmer for

about 1 hour, until the vegetables are soft and the peas are cooked through.

NUTRITIONAL INFORMATION PER SERVING

294 CALORIES • 13G PROTEIN • 4G FAT • 261MG SODIUM

VARIATION: You can substitute dried green peas for the yellow peas in this recipe.

TIP: Coconut cream can be made by combining one part water to four parts fresh, shredded coconut meat. Simmer the mixture until it foams. Strain it through a cheesecloth and be sure to squeeze out all the liquid.

## Lima Bean Soup with Smoked Turkey

As a kid, I remember seeing "old-timers" at Sylvia's ask for a bowl of lima beans with liquid—"Serve it soupy." That memory led me to create this recipe thirty years later. Fall and winter are the best times of the year for this nutritious, satisfying soup. It remains one of my family's favorite recipes.

*Serves 6*

2 smoked turkey legs

2 tablespoons olive oil

1 small onion, chopped

2 garlic cloves, minced

2 cups dried lima beans, soaked (page 103) and rinsed

2 quarts Easy Vegetable Stock (page 68)

## • NUTRITION COUNTS! •

I recently read that one of the directors at Harvard Medical School said American's lack of information about nutrition contributes both to disease and the out-of-control obesity rates. I learned this the hard way. You don't have to. Pay attention to the food you use, what goes in your stomach, and the size of the portions you eat.

2 teaspoons kosher salt
2 teaspoons fresh black pepper

1. Place the turkey in a pot and cover it with water. Bring to a boil and continue cooking for about 1 hour, until the meat is cooked and easily separates from the bone. Be sure the legs are always completely covered with water.
2. Take the legs out of the water and cut the meat from the bone. Place the meat in a large bowl and shred.* Set aside.
3. In a clean, large pot, heat the oil over high heat. Add the onions and garlic and cook for 3 to 5 minutes, until just starting to brown.
4. Add the turkey meat and stir well. Add the beans and stir well. Cook for 3 to 5 minutes. Add the vegetable stock and bring to a boil.
5. Lower the heat and simmer for 45 minutes, or until the beans are soft.

**NUTRITIONAL INFORMATION PER SERVING**
403 CALORIES • 32G PROTEIN • 13G FAT • 571MG SODIUM

*"Shred": Place meat, fish, or fowl in a bowl. Using two forks, pull the meat apart at the natural lines.

# Side Dishes

Most soul food meals come with a variety of sides. I'm not sure where this tradition comes from, but in Hemingway, South Carolina, while the men worked in the fields under the hot sun, the women cooked lots of dishes. That way, when the men returned, tired and hungry, they would have a full table of dishes to come home to.

Growing up, I loved macaroni and cheese and candied yams. But my all-time favorite side dish was one made by my great-grandma Julia in Hemingway. She made okra and butter beans like no one else. Grandma Sylvia says that Grandma Julia taught her how to cook, which is really saying something!

Soul food sides can be full of sugar, butter, or salt. If you find yourself eating a couple of side dishes, make sure your servings aren't too large. It's fun to sample a variety, but you don't want to overload yourself.

# Acorn Squash

To make citrus zesting easier, you can purchase a tool called a Microplane. They are available in the home department of many department stores as well as most hardware stores. *Serves 4*

1 tablespoon unsalted butter

2 tablespoons brown sugar, firmly packed

Juice of 1 orange

1 teaspoon grated nutmeg, plus extra for sprinkling

Grated zest of 1 orange

1 acorn squash, about 1 pound, halved and seeded

1. Preheat the oven to 350 degrees.
2. In a medium-sized saucepan, melt the butter and brown sugar and mix together well. Add the orange juice. Stir well and remove the pan from the heat. Whisk in the nutmeg, then add the orange zest.
3. Rub both halves of the squash with one-half of the butter mixture. Be sure to rub the flesh side as well as the skin side. Place the squash, flesh side down, on a baking sheet, and bake about 20 to 30 minutes, until it begins to soften.
4. With a pastry brush or barbecue brush, recoat the flesh side only of the squash with one-half of the remaining butter mixture and return the squash, flesh side down, to the baking sheet. Continue cooking for about 45 minutes, until the squash collapses in the center. Remove the sheet from the oven and let cool for about 10 minutes.

5. With a spoon, remove the flesh from the skin and place in a serving bowl. Reheat the remaining butter mixture and pour it over the squash. Mix well. Sprinkle with nutmeg and serve immediately.

VARIATION: You can also peel the entire squash and then cut it into cubes before baking. Place the cubes in a bowl and coat with the butter mixture. Place on a baking sheet and cook at 350 degrees until soft. Serve as a side dish similar to yams.

### NUTRITIONAL INFORMATION PER SERVING
214 CALORIES • 3G PROTEIN • 7G FAT • 74MG SODIUM

## Beulah's Best Beans

Beulah was my grandmother's sister, and she was responsible for carrying on many of my family's recipes, some of which would have been lost if not for her love of food and tradition.  *Serves 8*

1 tablespoon honey
2 tablespoons olive oil
2 sweet potatoes, peeled and cut into small cubes
1 pound string beans, washed, with ends trimmed
Salt and fresh black pepper to taste

1. Preheat the oven to 350 degrees.

2. In a large bowl, whisk together the honey, 1 tablespoon of the oil, and a pinch of salt. Add the sweet potatoes and toss.

3. Place the potatoes on a baking sheet and bake for 30 to 40 minutes, until they are soft. Remove from the oven and let cool slightly.

4. Heat the remaining tablespoon of oil in a large skillet. Add the string beans and sauté until the beans are soft and bright green. Remove the cooked beans from the skillet and let cool slightly.

5. In a large bowl, combine the potatoes and beans and toss until well combined. Season with salt and pepper to taste. Be sure to include any drippings or oil from the baking sheet or skillet.

**NUTRITIONAL INFORMATION PER SERVING**

157 CALORIES · 2G PROTEIN · 7G FAT · 8MG SODIUM

## Cornbread Stuffing

Cornmeal is a staple of many cultures, including ours. And you can't have an authentic soul food meal without stuffing. Here is a superb classic stuffing recipe featuring cornmeal.  *Serves 12*

Nonstick cooking spray

3 eggs, beaten

2 cups skim or lowfat milk

2 teaspoons kosher salt

6 tablespoons butter, melted

1 tablespoon baking powder

2½ cups cornmeal

1 teaspoon baking soda dissolved in 1 tablespoon water

1 onion, chopped

8 celery stalks, chopped

2 tablespoons dried sage

1 tablespoon chopped fresh parsley leaves

4 cups hot stock—chicken, turkey, or vegetable (see page 68)

Kosher salt and fresh black pepper to taste

1. Preheat the oven to 425 degrees. Spray an 8x8-inch square baking dish or similar dish with nonstick cooking spray.

2. In a large bowl, combine the eggs, milk, and salt and 3 tablespoons of the melted butter. Slowly add first the baking powder, then the cornmeal, to make a batter that resembles cake batter. (You might not need all of the cornmeal.) Beat the batter well. Add the baking soda water to the batter. Continue mixing.

3. Pour the batter into the prepared baking dish and bake for 20 to 25 minutes, until the bread begins to brown. Allow the bread to cool in the baking dish.

4. Break it into small pieces, crumbling the crust well.

5. Transfer the bread pieces to a large bowl and add the remaining 3 tablespoons of the melted butter and the onion, celery, sage, and parsley. Moisten with stock and season with salt and pepper. Stir well.

6. You can now fill your chicken or turkey. Or you can transfer the mixture to a 9x12-inch baking dish and bake at 350 degrees, until the top is brown and crispy.

TIP: If you like moist dressing, use a smaller baking dish and pile the bread higher before baking. For a crispier crust, spread the bread in a dish no more than 2 inches deep. These methods will alter your baking time, so watch the bread carefully so it does not burn.

NUTRITIONAL INFORMATION PER SERVING

210 CALORIES · 6G PROTEIN · 12G FAT · 403MG SODIUM

## Savory Brown Rice

Brown rice can be a healthy and delicious addition to so many dishes you prepare at home.

This recipe is for brown rice as a stand-alone side dish, rather than an accompaniment to a stew or other main dish.   *Serves 8*

1 tablespoon butter

1 tablespoon olive oil

1 onion, chopped

3 garlic cloves, minced

4 to 6 scallions, sliced

1 pound uncooked brown rice

4 teaspoons kosher salt

2 teaspoons fresh black pepper

½ bunch thyme, stripped (leaves only) (see page 33)

1 quart Easy Vegetable Stock
  (see page 68)

1. Heat the butter and olive oil in a large pot over high heat. Add the onion, garlic, and scallions and cook for 3 to 5 minutes, until soft.
2. Add the rice. Stir until it's well combined and the rice is shiny from the oil. Stir in the salt, pepper, thyme, and vegetable stock.
3. Cover the pot and lower the heat. Cook for 30 to 40 minutes, until the rice is cooked through.

NUTRITIONAL INFORMATION PER SERVING

100 CALORIES • 2G PROTEIN • 3G FAT • 113MG SODIUM

# • MATCH THE FLAVOR OF YOUR RICE TO YOUR MAIN PROTEIN •

If you are serving chicken, use chicken stock. If you are just looking for a neutral flavor, use vegetable stock. Or if you are serving beef, replace with beef stock. This is a good way to tie your meal together and keep the flavors compatible.

# Butter Beans and Okra

When I was growing up, this was actually one of the very few vegetable dishes I would eat. And the only person who made it exactly as I liked it was my great-grandmother Julia.   *Serves 6*

6 cups turkey or Easy Vegetable Stock (page 68)

1 pound smoked turkey legs

2 (10-ounce) packages frozen butter beans, thawed

1 tablespoon Mrs. Dash seasoning blend

2 teaspoons kosher salt

2 teaspoons fresh black pepper

2 cups fresh or frozen okra, chopped

1. In a large pot, bring the stock to a boil over a medium-high heat.
2. Add the turkey and reduce the heat. Simmer for 1½ hours, or until the turkey is soft.
3. Remove the turkey legs and let them cool slightly. Then remove the meat from bones and cut meat into small pieces. Return the meat to the pot.
4. Stir in the beans, Mrs. Dash, salt, and pepper and simmer for 15 to 20 minutes.
5. Stir in the okra and continue cooking for another 10 to 15 minutes, until the beans and okra are soft and the mixture is thickened.

**NUTRITIONAL INFORMATION PER SERVING**

284 CALORIES • 30G PROTEIN • 9G FAT • 457MG SODIUM

# Butternut Squash with Cinnamon and Pecans

All you carb lovers out there should know that squash is considered an excellent substitute for potatoes—with a fraction of the calories. *Serves 6*

2 tablespoons butter

1 tablespoon honey

2 teaspoons cinnamon

1 pound butternut squash, peeled, cleaned, and diced

8 ounces pecans, chopped

1. Preheat the oven to 350 degrees.

2. In a medium saucepan, melt the butter with the honey. Remove the pan from the heat and whisk in 1 teaspoon of the cinnamon. Set aside.

3. In a large bowl, combine the squash and the butter mixture. Use your hands to toss the mixture to be sure you are thoroughly combining the ingredients. Place the squash on a baking sheet and bake for 30 to 45 minutes, until the squash is soft. Remove the pan from the oven and let it cool for 5 minutes.

4. Transfer the squash to a large bowl and mix in the pecans using a rubber spatula.

5. Transfer to a serving bowl or platter and sprinkle the top with the remaining teaspoon of cinnamon.

### NUTRITIONAL INFORMATION PER SERVING

309 CALORIES · 4G PROTEIN · 68G FAT · 3MG SODIUM

## Country-Style Greens

Mustard and collard greens are vegetable staples in a soul food diet. Unfortunately, far too often in Southern cooking these healthy vegetables are cooked with pork, adding unnecessary calories and cholesterol. My grandmother's cousin, "Aunt" Coute, is the inspiration behind this great healthier recipe. *Serves 6*

1 pound mustard greens
1 pound collard greens

### · HOW LONG TO COOK GREENS ·

I have watched my mother and grandmother cook greens all day long. It all depends on how tough the greens are and if you cook them with the stalks, which lengthens the cooking time. Greens like collard, mustard, kale, and turnips are all sturdy vegetables and it takes a lot of time to break them down. Experienced cooks know it can be better to use your nose rather than your watch to tell when they are done. When the greens "perfume the air"—after a couple of hours—you know they are done.

2 to 3 tablespoons olive oil, to coat the bottom of the pot

1 onion, chopped

4 garlic cloves, chopped

1 smoked turkey wing, cut apart at the joints, or 2 smoked turkey
  necks

2 cups Easy Vegetable Stock (page 68)

2 teaspoons honey

½ teaspoon red pepper flakes

Kosher salt and pepper to taste

1. Take each bunch of green leaves, roll it like a cigar, and cut it crosswise
   into ribbons.

2. Fill a clean sink with cold water, place the cut greens in the sink, and
   rinse them well, agitating them with your hands to loosen the dirt and
   sand. (You may have to rinse them several times to get rid of all of the
   dirt.) Remove the greens and place them in a colander to drain.
   Remove from the top first, so the dirt on the bottom of the sink is not
   reintroduced into the clean greens.

3. Coat the bottom of a Dutch oven–style pot with the olive oil and sauté
   the onion and garlic over medium heat until they are soft. Add the
   smoked turkey and cook about 10 minutes, until the turkey begins to
   brown and release its juices.

4. Warm the broth, stir in the honey, and heat until it fully dissolves.

5. Add the greens to the turkey and stir until the greens are coated with
   oil and appear slick and shiny. Add enough broth mixture to just cover
   the greens. Reserve any leftover liquid for later use. Add the red pepper flakes.

6. Bring to a boil, then lower to a simmer. Cook until the greens are soft,
   about 1½ to 2½ hours. Season with salt and pepper to taste.

NUTRITIONAL INFORMATION PER SERVING

228 CALORIES · 11G PROTEIN · 9G FAT · 81MG SODIUM

Tɪᴘ: You can freeze your leftover broth in ice cube trays and then transfer cubes to freezer bags for easy access.

Tɪᴘ: Save any greens that you may not consume immediately to make Lenzo's Carolina Trout Stuffed with Collard Greens (page 121).

# D.R.'s Sweet Potatoes and Apples

Sweet potatoes and apples have long been soul food staples. D.R., my friend's mother, created this special blending of two of my favorites for a tremendous taste. Just remember to eat only an average-sized portion.
*Serves 8*

4 tablespoons butter

2 tablespoons honey

4 teaspoons cinnamon

Nonstick cooking spray

4 to 6 sweet potatoes, peeled and thinly sliced

10 apples of your favorite type, peeled, cored, and thinly sliced
   (slightly thicker than the potatoes)

1. Preheat the oven to 350 degrees.
2. Melt the butter with the honey in a medium saucepan over low heat. When melted, remove the pan from the heat and whisk in 2 teaspoons of the cinnamon.
3. Spray a 9x12-inch baking dish with nonstick cooking spray.
4. Make a layer of potato slices on the bottom of the dish, using half the potatoes. Then place a layer of apples on top of them. Drizzle the top with the butter mixture. Repeat the layering and top with the remaining 2 teaspoons cinnamon.
5. Bake for 30 to 35 minutes, or until the potatoes and apples are soft.

TIP: To ensure even slices with any fruit or vegetable, you may want to invest in a kitchen tool called a Benriner mandoline, or vegetable slicer. It is a Japanese tool that makes slicing a breeze! A Benriner comes with special attachments that allow you to do a variety of specialty cuts. When you prepare D.R.'s Sweet Potatoes and Apples, the adjustable blade will allow you to cut the apples slightly thicker than the potatoes to ensure even cooking. Be sure to read the directions thoroughly, and be cautious, because a Benriner is sharp. You may find it in Gracious Home, Williams-Sonoma, Broadway Panhandler, or similar stores.

**NUTRITIONAL INFORMATION PER SERVING**

390 CALORIES · 13G PROTEIN · 1G FAT · 17MG SODIUM

# Lenzo's Carolina Cabbage and Turkey Bacon

~~~~~~~~~~~

"Lenzo" is one of my favorite nicknames from childhood. And this cabbage dish is one of my all-time favorite vegetable recipes. Here I've added the turkey bacon for even more flavor.   *Serves 6*

> 6 strips turkey bacon
>
> 1 tablespoon olive oil
>
> 1 pound white cabbage, cored, chopped, and
>    washed
>
> 1½ cups Easy Vegetable Stock (page 68)
>    or water
>
> Salt and fresh black pepper
>    to taste

1. Heat the bacon in a medium-sized skillet over high heat and cook the strips until they are crisp. Remove the strips and drain them on a plate lined with paper towels. Save the skillet with the bacon drippings intact and add the oil. When the bacon is cool, finely chop (or crumble) the strips and set aside.

2. Place the cabbage in a colander. Put the vegetable stock in the bottom of a large pot that will house the colander. Cover the pot and colander and place it over high heat until the liquid begins to boil and you can see steam escaping from under the lid.

3. Lower the heat to prevent liquid from evaporating too quickly and

continue to cook the cabbage for 25 to 30 minutes, or until it's soft. Remove from the heat and let cool slightly.

4. In a large bowl, combine the cabbage, the oil and drippings from the skillet, and the bacon. Toss until well combined.

5. Season with salt and pepper to taste.

TIP: To clean cabbage, clean your sink and fill it with cold water. Cut the cabbage head crosswise into two halves. Cut the halves into quarters and remove the core. Cut each quarter crosswise into strips. Place the cut cabbage in the water and agitate it to remove all dirt. Cabbage heads grow with the leaves naturally held together so tightly that there is minimal dirt in between.

### NUTRITIONAL INFORMATION PER SERVING
145 CALORIES · 8G PROTEIN · 6G FAT · 299MG SODIUM

## Okra and Tomatoes

Okra is one of those vegetables that is abundant in the South. For generations it was a staple in most homes. This particular recipe is an excellent side dish, and I know many people enjoy it as a leftover for breakfast by adding some grits.   *Serves 4*

4 slices turkey bacon
1 tablespoon olive oil

1 small onion, chopped

1½ cups fresh okra, washed and cut into rounds

2 cups canned peeled tomatoes, crushed by hand

Salt and pepper to taste

1. Heat the bacon in a medium-sized pot and cook over high heat until crisp. Remove the bacon to a plate lined with paper towels. Let cool. Reserve the bacon drippings in the pot and add the oil.
2. When the bacon is cool, chop it and set it aside.
3. Reheat the same oil in the same pot and add the onion. Cook until soft. Add the okra and stir until they are combined. Add the tomatoes and stir to combine. Lower the heat and simmer until one-quarter of the liquid has evaporated and the mixture has thickened.
4. Add the chopped bacon. Season with salt and pepper to taste.

VARIATION: My grandmother used to add fresh sweet corn to this mix to add even more flavor. Try it by adding corn at step 3.

NUTRITIONAL INFORMATION PER SERVING

101 CALORIES · 6G PROTEIN · 7G FAT · 206MG SODIUM

# Red Beans and Rice

Peas and rice is a common Caribbean side dish, in which the peas are often pigeon peas or cowpeas. Here's my soul food version using red beans. *Serves 12*

2 tablespoons olive oil

2 tablespoons unsalted butter

1 onion, chopped

3 garlic cloves, chopped

1 bunch scallions, sliced

½ bunch fresh thyme, stripped (leaves only) (see page 33)

4 teaspoons kosher salt

2 teaspoons fresh black pepper

½ cup unsweetened coconut milk

8 ounces dried red beans, soaked and drained (see page 103)

1 pound uncooked white rice

1 quart Easy Vegetable Stock (page 68)

1. Heat the oil and butter in a large pot over high heat. Add the onion, garlic, and scallions and cook for 5 minutes, or until the ingredients are all soft.

2. Add the thyme leaves, salt, pepper, and coconut milk. Stir until they are all combined. Continue cooking for 3 to 5 minutes to release flavors.

3. Add the beans and rice and stir until well combined. Add the vegetable stock and stir again. Then bring it all to a boil.

4. Cook over a very low flame for 45 minutes, until the rice is cooked through and the beans are soft. Be sure to add more stock as needed in order to keep the rice and the beans moist.

**NUTRITIONAL INFORMATION PER SERVING**

288 CALORIES · 10G PROTEIN · 6G FAT · 317MG SODIUM

# Shon Gables's Stovetop Squash Casserole

Shon Gables is co-anchor of CBS 2 News' "This Morning in New York." She has received numerous media and journalism awards. Thanks, Shon, for sharing your casserole recipe.    *Serves 4*

⅓ cup olive oil or vegetable oil

6 whole yellow squash, sliced

1 large onion, diced

6 slices bacon, turkey bacon, or lowfat bacon, pan-fried and diced

1 tablespoon salt

1 tablespoon fresh black pepper

1 tablespoon minced garlic (optional)

Shredded lowfat cheddar cheese (optional)

1. Heat the oil in a large pan on medium-high heat.
2. Combine the squash slices, onion, bacon, salt, pepper, and garlic in a medium mixing bowl and add the mixture to the pan.

3. Cover the pan with a lid and simmer for 20 minutes, until the squash is soft. Remove and let cool.

4. Lightly sprinkle with lowfat cheddar cheese, if desired.

CAUTION: Do not add water—squash makes its own liquid, and it's delicious!

NUTRITIONAL INFORMATION PER SERVING

349 CALORIES · 10G PROTEIN · 24G FAT · 718MG SODIUM

## Rice Noodles and Peppers

Fresh peppers and onions add a tangy taste to so many dishes. This recipe can be enjoyed as a meal—just add a salad—or as a side dish for chicken or beef. *Serves 8*

1 pound rice noodles

1 tablespoon sesame oil

1 red onion, sliced

1 red pepper, julienned

1 yellow pepper, julienned

2 cups soy sauce

Fresh black pepper

1. Prepare the noodles according to the package directions.
2. Heat the oil in a large skillet or wok over high heat. Add the onion and peppers. Cook about 5 minutes, until vegetables are softened.
3. Add the rice noodles and soy sauce to the skillet. Toss to combine, then simmer for 6 to 8 minutes.
4. Remove from the heat and sprinkle with black pepper.

**NUTRITIONAL INFORMATION PER SERVING**

312 CALORIES · 9G PROTEIN · 7G FAT · 1176MG SODIUM

## Vegetable Fried Rice

Knowing how to prepare a "well" is part of this recipe. Here's how: Using a rubber spatula and the sides of your pan, push the contents up and toward the edges to create a space in the middle. Woks have unusually high sides just for this purpose. Do not be concerned if you cannot move all the contents out of the way. Even a small space will do the trick.

*Serves 6*

1 pound brown rice

½ cup sesame oil or peanut oil

1 large onion, cut into small dice

4 celery stalks, cut into small dice

2 carrots, peeled and cut into small dice

1 tablespoon minced ginger

1 yellow pepper, cut into small dice

1 red pepper, cut into small dice

1-pound package bamboo shoots

1 bunch scallions, sliced

¼ cup soy sauce

2 tablespoons sesame seeds

1. Cook the rice according to the package directions and set aside.
2. Heat a large skillet or wok over high heat and add the oil. When the oil begins to smoke, add the onion, celery, carrot, ginger, yellow pepper, and red pepper. Cook for 3 to 5 minutes, until the vegetables are tender.
3. Add the rice and toss until the mixture is well combined. Add the bamboo shoots, scallions, and soy sauce. Toss again.
4. Lower the heat and simmer the mixture for 5 to 8 minutes, until the flavors combine.
5. Remove from the heat and toss the rice with the sesame seeds. Serve immediately.

VARIATION: Scramble 4 to 6 egg whites or the equivalent egg substitute in a "well" just before you remove from heat. This is a classic Asian ingredient. You can also mix it up with a combination of black and white sesame seeds.

NUTRITIONAL INFORMATION PER SERVING

96 CALORIES · 9G PROTEIN · 11G FAT · 321MG SODIUM

# Macaroni and Cheese

You can't have a soul food cookbook without a recipe for macaroni and cheese. Is it possible, you may ask, for mac and cheese to be healthy *and* delicious? Yes, it is! Try this recipe and see.  *Serves 8*

1 pound elbow macaroni
2 tablespoons butter
2 tablespoons whole-wheat or unbleached flour
1½ pints skim milk
1 cup shredded cheddar cheese
1 cup shredded Monterey jack cheese
1 cup shredded mozzarella cheese
Nonstick cooking spray

1. Cook the macaroni according to the package directions, but subtract 3 or 4 minutes from the cooking time. The macaroni should be a bit underdone, since it will cook a second time. Drain and set aside.
2. Preheat the oven to 350 degrees.
3. In a large saucepan, melt the butter. When it begins to brown, add the flour and whisk until combined. Cook until you can smell the butter/flour combination, 6 to 8 minutes.
4. While continuing to whisk, begin to add milk gradually until you have a cream sauce. You may need to add more if the sauce seems too thick.
5. Once the cream sauce is thin enough, begin to add the cheeses while continuing to whisk. Again you may need more milk to thin your

sauce. Continue this process while whisking until all the cheese is melted in.

6. Remove from the heat and fold in the macaroni. Spray a casserole dish with nonstick cooking spray and pour the mixture into the dish.

7. Bake for 35 to 40 minutes, until the macaroni is heated through and brown on top.

VARIATION: To lower the fat content, you can substitute lowfat or part-skim cheeses for regular cheese.

**NUTRITIONAL INFORMATION PER SERVING**

422 CALORIES · 28G PROTEIN · 29G FAT · 470MG SODIUM

# Entrées

I'm proud of my African-American heritage, and proud of African-American food. The whole point of this book is to find a way to eat our food in a healthier way. This is especially important for soul food entrées.

Soul food meals can include a variety of entrées, but I generally only allow myself one, about 4 to 5 ounces per meal. That might not sound like a lot, but if you cook your entrée right, it can be satisfying and filling.

You don't need to make complicated entrées either. One of my favorite entrées is pepper chicken, cooked skinless in olive oil and only coated with pepper. It's a simple dish, and that's what makes it so good. When you buy quality organic ingredients, you don't always need to cover them with fancy sauces or too much preparation. When I do use a sauce,

I try to keep it healthy, with as few preservatives or additives as possible. For example, I sometimes put some peaches in a skillet and simmer them until they melt into a sauce. If you pour this sauce over a chicken leg and thigh—the juiciest part of the chicken—and let it cook, then you're preparing a healthy, tasty dish with a minimum of fuss.

## Lemon and Garlic Tofu

I bet you didn't know that soy has 75 percent less fat than beef. If you haven't tried soy products—including tofu—you will be surprised at the taste and versatility.    *Serves 4*

½ stick butter

¼ cup olive oil

1 pound firm tofu, drained, dried, and cut into medium dice

1 garlic clove, minced

Grated zest and juice of 1 lemon

2 teaspoons kosher salt

1 teaspoon fresh black pepper

1 cup Easy Vegetable Stock (page 68)

1 teaspoon chopped fresh parsley, for garnish

1. In a large skillet, heat the butter and olive oil over high heat. Add the tofu and cook 5 to 8 minutes, until brown.

2. Add the garlic, lemon zest, lemon juice, salt, pepper, and stock. Simmer for 15 to 20 minutes.

3. Garnish with the parsley before serving.

**NUTRITIONAL INFORMATION PER SERVING**

630 CALORIES · 40G PROTEIN · 48G FAT · 999MG SODIUM

# Eggplant Parmigiana

Aunt Coute had the best eggplant recipe, North or South, bar none. It was so good we only needed to change a few ingredients to make it delicious and healthy.  *Serves 8*

2 cups tomato sauce

2 egg whites

1 cup wheat germ, ground in a coffee grinder or food processor

2 teaspoons dried thyme

2 teaspoons dried oregano

1 teaspoon kosher salt

1 teaspoon fresh black pepper

1 large eggplant, peeled, sliced lengthwise into ½-inch slices, and
    purged (see Note)

Nonstick cooking spray

1 pound skim-milk mozzarella, shredded

1. Heat the tomato sauce in a medium saucepan over low heat just long enough to warm it. Set aside.

2. Place the egg whites in a large platter. Mix the wheat germ, thyme, oregano, salt, and pepper in a bowl, then transfer it to a second platter or dish. Dip the eggplant slices in the egg whites, then in the wheat germ coating. Repeat with each eggplant slice until all are coated.

3. Preheat the oven to 350 degrees.

4. Spray a large skillet with nonstick cooking spray and place it over medium-high heat. Add the eggplant slices and fry until crispy on both sides. Drain on a plate lines with paper towels.

5. Spoon enough of the tomato sauce into a 9x12-inch baking dish to cover the bottom. Add a layer of eggplant, then sprinkle about half the cheese on top. Repeat until the eggplant is used up, ending with a topping of cheese.

6. Bake for about 45 minutes, until heated through and the cheese on top is melted.

NOTE: To purge the eggplant, slice it and place it on a baking sheet lined with paper towels. Sprinkle with salt on both sides and cover with paper towels. Let the slices sit for at least two hours. Blot dry before using. This "purging" process removes excess water from the eggplant, which results in a crispier product.

NUTRITIONAL INFORMATION PER SERVING

250 CALORIES · 21G PROTEIN · 10G FAT · 370MG SODIUM

## Okra Gumbo

~~~~~~~~

I grew up on okra gumbo, but I wish I had this healthy version way back then. This is an update of my family's traditional gumbo.   *Serves 6*

¼ cup olive oil

1 onion, cut into small dice

2 tablespoons brown sugar, firmly packed

2 quarts Easy Vegetable Stock (page 68)

2 teaspoons kosher salt

2 teaspoons fresh black pepper

2 cups okra, fresh or frozen, cut into thin rounds

2 cups whole-kernel corn, fresh or frozen

### · HOW TO SOAK BEANS ·

When using dry beans, you must either soak them overnight or use the quick-soak method.

To soak beans overnight, place them in a large deep bowl or plastic container. Cover with water to 2 inches above the bean line and soak overnight. The quick-soak method works this way: Place the beans in a large pot and cover them with water to 2 inches above bean line. Bring to a boil and then remove from the heat. Let the beans stand for 1½ hours. Rinse under cold water until the water runs clear. Use as desired.

1. Heat the oil in a large pot. Add the onion and cook until soft. Add the brown sugar and cook for 3 minutes. Add the stock and bring to a boil. Add the salt and pepper.

2. Add the okra and corn. Cover, reduce the heat, and simmer for 30 to 40 minutes.

VARIATION: For those of you who like meat or fish in your gumbo, try adding chorizo, andouille sausage, chicken, or shrimp, just after adding the brown sugar, for added flavor and substance.

**NUTRITIONAL INFORMATION PER SERVING**

283 CALORIES • 6G PROTEIN • 22G FAT • 34MG SODIUM

## Spinach Lasagna

I've talked a lot about helping our kids to eat right, be healthy, and not become one of the statistics of overweight kids. It's shocking to learn that 25 percent of children in this country are considered obese. I was one of them. Serving modified recipes, like this one for lasagna (and all the kids I know love lasagna), will help eliminate some of the fat in your family's diet.

*Serves 8*

1 pound lasagna noodles, cooked according to package directions
¼ cup olive oil
1 small onion, chopped
3 garlic cloves, minced
1 pound ground turkey

2 cups tomato sauce

2 1-pound bags of baby spinach, blanched, shocked, drained, and
chopped

1 pound lowfat cottage cheese, puréed

1 teaspoon kosher salt

1 teaspoon fresh black pepper

2 teaspoons grated nutmeg

1 pound lowfat mozzarella, shredded

1. Preheat the oven to 350 degrees. Prepare the lasagna noodles according to the package directions (preferably al dente). Set aside.

2. In a large skillet, heat the oil. Add the onion and garlic and cook until
soft. Add one-third of the turkey, crumbling the meat with a wooden
spoon or spatula. Continue cooking until the meat is cooked through.
Remove from the heat.

3. In a medium saucepan, heat the tomato sauce over low heat. Add
another third of the remaining turkey to the sauce. Stir and keep the
sauce warm over very low heat.

4. In a large bowl, combine the remaining turkey and the raw spinach,
cottage cheese, salt, pepper, and nutmeg.

5. Spoon enough meat sauce into a 9x12-inch baking dish to cover the bottom. Add a layer of noodles, then the spinach mixture, and then the
shredded mozzarella. Continue layering, ending with mozzarella on top.

6. Bake for 25 to 30 minutes, until the cheese is melted and the lasagna is
heated through. Remove from the oven. Let stand for 10 to 15 minutes to allow for easier cutting.

### NUTRITIONAL INFORMATION PER SERVING

700 CALORIES · 44G PROTEIN · 32G FAT · 358MG SODIUM

# Vegetable Croquettes

~~~~~~~~~~~~~~~~~~~~~

You probably know that any type of dried bean will absorb large amounts of water and salt. Always be sure that during the cooking process you check periodically to make sure there is enough water in the pot. In addition, taste-test your recipe for saltiness during cooking.   *Serves 8*

4 cups dried lentils

1 red pepper, diced

1 green pepper, diced

1 tablespoon dried thyme

1 garlic clove, minced

4 to 6 scallions, sliced

1 cup fresh breadcrumbs

2 teaspoons kosher salt

2 teaspoons fresh black pepper

¼ cup olive oil

1. Soak the beans overnight or use the quick-soak method (see page 103).
2. Rinse the lentils until the water runs clear.
3. Place the lentils in a large pot and cover them with water. Cook for 20 to 30 minutes, until they are soft. You may need to add water if they start to look dry. Drain the lentils completely and transfer to a large bowl. Add the red and green peppers, thyme, garlic, scallions, breadcrumbs, salt, and pepper and mix until thoroughly combined.
4. Using a tablespoon to measure out a small amount, roll the mixture into small balls and slightly flatten them.

5. In a large skillet, heat the oil over medium heat and fry the croquettes in batches for 10 to 15 minutes, or until both sides are browned.

### NUTRITIONAL INFORMATION PER SERVING

301 CALORIES · 44G PROTEIN · 33G FAT · 70MG SODIUM

## Down-Home Hot Shrimp Stew

This dish is a lot like gumbo. It tastes best when it's made just a little hot and spicy. *Serves 6*

3 tablespoons olive oil
1 garlic clove, minced

## · SHRIMP STOCK ·

Tip: Save the shrimp shells and use them to make stock for the stew. Heat 2 tablespoons olive oil in a large pot. Cook 1 sliced onion until soft. Add 1 carrot and 4 stalks of celery, cut into large dice. Add 1 cup of white wine. Cook, stirring, until reduced by half. Add 4 quarts of water, 3 or 4 bay leaves, and a handful of black peppercorns and bring to a boil. Reduce the heat and let the stock simmer until the liquid reduces again by half, which takes about 2 to 3 hours.

1 onion, sliced

6 celery stalks, chopped

2 red peppers, sliced

2 yellow peppers, sliced

2 orange peppers, sliced

2 tablespoons whole-wheat flour

1 cup shrimp stock (see page 107)

2 teaspoons Mrs. Dash seasoning blend

1 teaspoon kosher salt

2 teaspoons fresh black pepper

1 tablespoon crushed red pepper flakes

1 large Idaho potato, peeled and cubed

2 cups canned tomatoes, crushed by hand

1 pound medium shrimp, peeled and deveined

1. Heat the oil in a large pot over high heat. Add the garlic, onion, and celery and all the sliced peppers. Stir and cook for 3 minutes until soft. Add the flour and stir until well combined.
2. Add the stock, Mrs. Dash, salt, black pepper, and red pepper flakes. Bring to a boil and stir in the potato and tomatoes.
3. Bring to a second boil, stir, and reduce the heat to a simmer. Simmer for 40 minutes. Add the shrimp and cook for another 5 minutes.

NUTRITIONAL INFORMATION PER SERVING

412 CALORIES · 14G PROTEIN · 18G FAT · 99MG SODIUM

# Shrimp Stew

Don't be afraid to experiment in the kitchen. I've made a career out of blending the old with the new, and the results have been powerful. When preparing this shrimp stew, if you prefer other vegetables or want to omit a spice—be my guest. Great chefs know that being flexible and daring yields excellent results.    *Serves 4*

2 tablespoons olive oil

1 onion, cut into small dice

3 garlic cloves, minced

2 celery stalks, cut into small dice

2 carrots, peeled and cut into small dice

3 potatoes, peeled and cut into small dice

2 teaspoons paprika

1 teaspoon cayenne pepper

2 teaspoons kosher salt

2 teaspoons fresh black pepper

2 quarts shrimp stock (see page 107)

1 pound medium shrimp, peeled and deveined

1. In a large pot, heat the oil over high heat. Add the onion and garlic and cook until soft.
2. Add the celery, carrots, and potatoes. Cook, stirring, until they start to soften, about 7 to 8 minutes.
3. Stir in the paprika, cayenne, salt, and pepper. Add the stock and simmer until the potatoes are tender, about 10 to 15 minutes.

4. Stir in the shrimp and cook about an additional 10 minutes, until the shrimp are pink and curled.

NUTRITIONAL INFORMATION PER SERVING

205 CALORIES • 23G PROTEIN • 11G FAT • 188MG SODIUM

## Ed Bradley's Shrimp Creole

Ed Bradley is the legendary *60 Minutes* reporter—and a longtime Sylvia's customer. He generously shares his favorite shrimp dish here in *Neo Soul*.
*Serves 8*

¾ stick unsalted butter

2½ cups finely chopped onions

2 teaspoons finely minced garlic

1 cup chopped celery

3 green bell peppers, chopped into ¾-inch pieces

2 jalapeño peppers, seeded and minced

Salt and fresh black pepper to taste

4 cups cubed tomatoes

¼ cup finely chopped parsley leaves

1 bay leaf

1 tablespoon Matouk's Hot Sauce, or to taste (optional)
  (see Note)

2 pounds medium shrimp, peeled and deveined
Rice and lemon wedges, for serving

1. Heat 2 tablespoons of the butter in a saucepan over medium heat and sauté the onions and garlic for 5 minutes. Do not brown.
2. Add the celery, bell peppers, and jalapeños to the pan and season with salt and pepper to taste. Cook for about 4 minutes, stirring often. Do not let the vegetables become soggy; they should remain crisp.
3. Add the tomatoes, parsley, and bay leaf. Cover and bring to a boil. Simmer for 10 minutes and stir in the Matouk's sauce. Remove the bay leaf.
4. Heat the remaining 4 tablespoons of the butter in a frying pan over high heat and sauté the shrimp for 1 minute. Pour the tomato mixture over the shrimp, stir well, and bring just to a boil. Remove from the heat and serve with rice and lemon wedges.

NOTE: Matouk's hot sauce, a fiery blend of papaya and hot peppers from Trinidad, is available in some West Indian and Indian shops, including in Manhattan—West Side Gourmet, 2528 Broadway, and K. Kalustvan (where it is also available by mail), 123 Lexington Avenue, New York, NY, 10016. This is not Matouk's hot *pepper* sauce, which is probably too hot for this dish.

**NUTRITIONAL INFORMATION PER SERVING**

262 CALORIES · 25G PROTEIN · 11G FAT · 198MG SODIUM

# • MY CELEBRITY PALS' FAVORITE SOUL FOOD MEALS •

- LL Cool J: LL is a traditional soul food kind of guy—he always has the fried chicken, the macaroni and cheese, and the collard greens.
- Taye Diggs: Taye has lots of favorites, but he particularly loves Red Velvet Cake from Sylvia's. (See my version on page 161).
- Latrell Sprewell: Latrell eats pretty healthy and likes organic food. He loves Seafood Alfredo Pasta and Banana Pudding, a soul food favorite.
- Ed Bradley: Ed is known as the Collard Greens Man! Check out Mr. Bradley's Shrimp Creole recipe on page 110.
- Russell Simmons: Russell used to scarf down barbecued ribs, macaroni and cheese, and collard greens, but recently he's become a vegan. So it's only the vegetables for him!
- Chris Rock: Chris told me loud and clear that he loves fried chicken, mac and cheese, and yams.
- Alicia Keys: Fillet of Sole on a bed of rice . . . sweet Southern-style.
- The Reverend Al and Mrs. Sharpton: These wonderful people are two of Sylvia's regulars. When they take out, grilled chicken salad and fried potatoes extra crispy!
- Shon Gables: Shon, a CBS 2 Morning News anchor, is a talented, beautiful breath of fresh air here in New York City. She shares her own special soul food casserole dish on page 92.

# Broiled Flounder

Here's something I read recently about fish: Research shows that older women with clogged coronary arteries who eat at least two servings of fish a week can slow the progression of atherosclerosis. Of course, fish is healthy for the entire family.    *Serves 4*

4 flounder fillets

2 teaspoons garlic powder

2 teaspoons kosher salt

2 teaspoons fresh black pepper

1 tablespoon Mrs. Dash seasoning blend

2 cups whole-wheat flour

1. Preheat the broiler.
2. Dry the fish with paper towels and set aside.
3. In a small bowl, combine the garlic powder, salt, pepper, and Mrs. Dash. Mix until well combined. Sprinkle the spice mixture on both sides of the fillets.
4. Place the flour in a platter and coat each fillet. Discard any unused flour.
5. Place the fillets in the broiling pan or equivalent and place in the broiler. Broil 3 to 5 minutes on each side, depending on the thickness of the fillets.

### NUTRITIONAL INFORMATION PER SERVING

217 CALORIES · 38G PROTEIN · 3G FAT · 93MG SODIUM

# Roasted Red Snapper

I recall many a family Labor Day party in South Carolina where red snapper was on the menu. I use fish in many of my recipes for catering and parties today, and snapper is a healthy, delicious favorite.   *Serves 10*

1 teaspoon Mrs. Dash seasoning blend

2 teaspoons kosher salt

2 teaspoons fresh black pepper

2 bunches fresh thyme, stripped (leaves only) (see page 33)

2 cups olive oil

4 pounds red snapper fillets

1. Preheat the oven to 325 degrees.
2. In a small bowl, combine the Mrs. Dash, salt, pepper, thyme leaves, and oil. Brush both sides of each fillet with the oil mixture. Place the fillets on a baking sheet and bake for 20 to 30 minutes, basting every 10 minutes. The fish is completely cooked when it becomes flaky and starts to brown.
3. Remove the baking sheet from the oven and let the fish cool slightly before serving.

### NUTRITIONAL INFORMATION PER SERVING
421 CALORIES • 19G PROTEIN • 19G FAT • 199MG SODIUM

# Barbecued Salmon

~~~~~~~~~~~~~~~~~~~~~~

Barbecued food is a soul food classic. Here is my healthy updated spin on barbecue. This combines the flavor of barbecue with the healthy properties of salmon. You can't go wrong. *Serves 4*

¼ cup honey

6 garlic cloves, minced

2 cups tomato sauce

1½ cups tomato paste

1 tablespoon onion powder

1 teaspoon dry mustard

3 teaspoons kosher salt

3 teaspoons fresh black pepper

1 cup apple cider vinegar

1 pound salmon fillets, cut into 4 pieces

1 teaspoon Mrs. Dash seasoning blend

1. Preheat the grill.
2. In a medium saucepan, combine the honey and garlic over moderate heat and cook until the garlic begins to brown and soften.
3. Add the tomato sauce, tomato paste, onion powder, and mustard. Add 2 teaspoons of the salt and 2 teaspoons of the pepper. Mix until completely combined.
4. Add the vinegar and continue stirring. Bring to a boil and reduce the heat. Simmer for 6 to 8 minutes and then set aside.

5. Season the fish with the Mrs. Dash, the remaining 1 teaspoon salt, and the remaining 1 teaspoon pepper.

6. Place the salmon on the grill and cook 2 to 3 minutes per side. Remove from the heat, brush with the sauce, and serve.

NUTRITIONAL INFORMATION PER SERVING

460 CALORIES • 33G PROTEIN • 8G FAT • 750MG SODIUM

# Grilled Catfish

This tasty freshwater fish, once known only in the South, is now one of America's favorite fish. It has a tough skin that can be difficult to remove, so it's easier to buy fillets to prepare this recipe.   *Serves 4*

4 catfish fillets, about ½ inch thick

1 tablespoon Mrs. Dash seasoning blend

⅛ teaspoon salt

⅛ teaspoon fresh black pepper

Greated zest of 1 lemon

2 tablespoons olive oil

2 lemon wedges, for serving

Chopped parsley, for garnish

1. Preheat the grill. Whether you have a gas, electric, or charcoal grill, make sure that you get the fire going well before you begin to prepare the fish.

2. Dry the fish with paper towels and set aside.

3. Combine the Mrs. Dash, salt, pepper, zest, and olive oil in a plastic bag and shake well. Add the fish to the bag and shake it again. Make sure that the fish is adequately covered with the spice mixture.

4. Check to be sure that your grill is very hot. Coals or the equivalent should be glowing red-orange. Place the fish on the grill and listen for the sound of the fish being seared. This will confirm that your grill is hot enough. Leave the fish on one side for a full 3 minutes. *Do not move it or try to change the position.* This will disturb the cooking process and the fish will begin to fall apart.

5. After 3 minutes, turn the fish onto the other side and cook for another 3 minutes. Use a thin-bladed, long-handled spatula to turn the fish. (Tongs or a barbecue fork could cause the fish to break.)

6. Once the fish has begun to firm up, you might want to adjust the cooking time to avoid undercooked fish. You can tell that the fish is done when it flakes easily. Check with a fork, or remove the fish from the grill and check by lightly poking it with your finger.

7. When the fish is done, remove it from the grill. Top with juice from the lemon wedges and garnish with chopped parsley.

VARIATION: You can also broil this fish by using the same preparation method. Preheat your broiler to about 450 to 500 degrees and place the fish on the broiling pan. Broil for 3 to 5 minutes and then check for doneness as described in step 6. Adjust for additional time as needed.

NUTRITIONAL INFORMATION PER SERVING

78 CALORIES · 13G PROTEIN · 3G FAT · 76MG SODIUM

# Catfish Stew

*Serves 4*

1 (14-ounce) can whole peeled tomatoes

4 catfish fillets, cut into bite-sized pieces

1 teaspoon Mrs. Dash seasoning blend

½ teaspoon fresh black pepper

2 tablespoons olive oil

1 small onion, chopped

4 celery stalks, chopped

1 orange, red, or yellow pepper, chopped

2 tablespoons tomato paste

½ cup fish stock

½ cup tomato sauce

2 tablespoons honey

1 teaspoon paprika

2 teaspoons cayenne pepper

1. Rinse the tomatoes and place them in a large bowl. Squeeze the tomatoes in between your fingers so that they break apart. This allows you to control the size of the pieces so they are not too big. Set aside.

2. Dry the fish with paper towels. Season it with the Mrs. Dash and black pepper. Set aside.

3. Heat the oil over medium-high heat in a stew pot. Add the onion, celery, and chopped pepper. Cook until the vegetables are soft. Stir in the tomato paste and add the fish stock.

4. Bring to a boil and reduce the heat to low. Add the tomatoes, tomato

sauce, honey, paprika, and cayenne. Simmer for 8 to 10 minutes, until some of the liquid has evaporated.

5. Add the fish pieces and continue cooking for another 10 to 12 minutes, or until the fish is cooked through.

**NUTRITIONAL INFORMATION PER SERVING**

376 CALORIES · 28G PROTEIN · 25G FAT · 500MG SODIUM

## Tartar Sauce

Here's a quick little recipe for your own tartar sauce that's simple to prepare and much healthier than the bottled product. *Serves 12*

- ½ cup diced sour gherkins
- ¼ cup India Relish
- ¾ cup lowfat mayo
- 2 tablespoons chopped fresh parsley leaves
- 1 teaspoon fresh lemon juice
- ½ teaspoon grated lemon zest
- 1 teaspoon fennel seeds or celery seeds
- ½ teaspoon honey

In a medium bowl, combine all the ingredients and mix well. Cover and refrigerate immediately. Chill the sauce for at least one hour for maximum flavor. Serve it with Codfish Cakes (page 120) or a similar fish entrée.

**NUTRITIONAL INFORMATION PER SERVING**

**(1 SERVING = 2 TABLESPOONS)**

88 CALORIES · 0G PROTEIN · 2G FAT · 159MG SODIUM

# Codfish Cakes

Fish cakes are the perfect food to prepare and freeze for later use. After you have formed all of the fish cakes, lay them on a baking sheet, cover, and freeze. Once they're frozen, you can transfer them to freezer bags. This way you can take out as many as you need, when you need them.

*Serves 4*

1 Idaho potato, peeled and cut into cubes

2 pounds codfish fillets, soaked in cold water for at least 2 hours, dried with paper towels and cut into cubes

1 red pepper, cut into small dice

1 green pepper, cut into small dice

1 garlic clove, minced

4 to 6 scallions, sliced

4 egg whites

1 cup fresh breadcrumbs

2 teaspoons kosher salt

2 teaspoons fresh black pepper

½ cup olive oil

Tartar Sauce, for serving (page 119)

1. Place the potato in a small pot and cover it with water. Cook over high heat until very soft. Then drain, mash, and set aside.

2. Place the fish in a food processor and grind until there are no more large pieces. If you do not own a food processor, you can mince the

fish with your knife. Just make sure that the cod resembles cooked oatmeal before going to the next step.

3. Transfer the cod to a large bowl. Fold in the mashed potato, peppers, garlic, scallions, egg whites, breadcrumbs, salt, and pepper. Mix well until all the ingredients are combined. Form the entire mixture into small (¼-cup) cakes.

4. Put enough oil in a large skillet to cover the bottom and place it over medium-high heat. When the skillet is hot, cook the cakes in batches, about 5 minutes per side, until they are brown on both sides and cooked through.

5. Serve with Tartar Sauce (page 119).

TIP: If you make the fish cakes in advance and freeze them, they can go into the skillet with minimal defrosting.

### NUTRITIONAL INFORMATION PER SERVING

512 CALORIES • 21G PROTEIN • 59G FAT • 197MG SODIUM

## Lenzo's Carolina Trout Stuffed with Collard Greens

In preparing this dish you will need cooking twine. You can buy it in most kitchen and cooking stores. (Just be sure you use it for cooking only.) Don't be afraid of a new spin on an old familiar dish. Never had trout prepared this way? Then you're in for a treat. *Serves 4*

4 trout fillets, about ½ inch thick

4 cups collard greens (see page 84)

1 onion, chopped fine

6 garlic cloves, chopped fine

1 teaspoon crushed red pepper flakes

Grated zest of 1 lemon

⅛ teaspoon salt

⅛ teaspoon fresh black pepper

3 egg whites

2 teaspoons Mrs. Dash seasoning blend

Nonstick cooking spray

1. Dry the fillets with paper towels and set aside.
2. To squeeze water from the greens, place them in a colander in the sink and press out the water. Or place them in a thin cloth towel or cheese-cloth and squeeze the water into a bowl or over the sink. This method would require the process to be done in 1½-cup batches.
3. Chop the greens fine, so that there are no large stems or pieces. They should resemble chopped spinach.
4. Place the greens, onion, garlic, red pepper flakes, lemon zest, salt, pepper, and egg whites in a large bowl and mix well. The mixture should hold together by itself.
5. Preheat the oven to 350 degrees.
6. Season the fish on all sides with the Mrs. Dash. Place one fillet at a time in front of you, head or tail at 12 o'clock and the other end at 6 o'clock, and place the filling down the center of the fillet, leaving about a ½-inch to 1-inch space at each end. Rolling away from you, roll the fillet together with the filling. Secure the fillet with cooking twine if you like. Spray a

9x12-inch baking dish with nonstick cooking spray and place the fish seam side down. Repeat for all the fillets.

7. Bake the fish 40 minutes.

**NUTRITIONAL INFORMATION PER SERVING**
246 CALORIES · 29G PROTEIN · 3G FAT · 73MG SODIUM

## Chicken and Vegetables in Tomato Sauce

This is a meal the whole family will love, and it's loaded with good foods.

*Serves 8*

2 cups olive oil

1 onion, cut into small dice

1 (10-ounce) package of frozen mixed vegetables

1 red pepper, cut into small dice

1 orange pepper, cut into small dice

2 pounds skinless, boneless chicken breasts, cut into large dice

1 quart chicken stock

2 cups tomato sauce

2 tablespoons honey

1 teaspoon kosher salt

1 teaspoon fresh black pepper

1. Heat the oil in a large pot over high heat. Add the onion and cook until soft. Add the frozen vegetables, red and orange peppers, and chicken pieces. Cook, stirring, 10 to 12 minutes, until the vegetables begin to soften and the chicken begins to brown.

2. Add the chicken stock. Continue stirring until some of the liquid evaporates, about 6 to 8 minutes.

3. Add the tomato sauce, honey, salt, and pepper. Stir and bring to a boil. Reduce the heat and continue to cook for about 30 minutes, until the chicken is tender and the vegetables are soft.

NUTRITIONAL INFORMATION PER SERVING

340 CALORIES • 30G PROTEIN • 58G FAT • 577MG SODIUM

## Mom's Broiled Chicken

Mom Bedelia is known as the family cook, and she always keeps her kitchen stocked in case family or friends drop by. This updated grilled chicken recipe has a couple of my mother's own unique ingredients plus my *Neo* spin.   *Serves 6*

2 pounds skinless, boneless chicken breasts

2 tablespoons olive oil

2 teaspoons Mrs. Dash seasoning blend

¼ cup Dijon mustard

2 tablespoons balsamic vinegar

Juice of 2 lemons

2 garlic cloves, minced

1. Preheat the oven to broil.
2. Pound the chicken with a kitchen mallet until it is flattened, being careful not to pound holes in it.
3. In a large plastic bag, combine the oil, Mrs. Dash, mustard, vinegar, lemon juice, and garlic. Shake well to combine.
4. Place the breasts in the bag two at a time and shake to coat the chicken. Continue until all the breasts are coated.
5. Place the breasts on the broiler pan in the oven. Cook for a total of 12 minutes, brushing the chicken every 2 minutes with the remaining sauce and turning it over.
6. Remove from the oven and let cool slightly before serving.

### NUTRITIONAL INFORMATION PER SERVING

180 CALORIES · 29G PROTEIN · 3G FAT · 66MG SODIUM

## Oven-Fried Chicken

*Serves 6*

2 teaspoons dried thyme

2 teaspoons dried oregano

2 teaspoons dried basil

2 teaspoons garlic powder

Exercising is probably the best thing you can do *right now* to get in better shape. Americans of all races tend to be less active than their grandparents were. The combination of fatty foods with little exercise equals the obesity epidemic we have today in the U.S.A. Fried chicken is such a central component of Southern cooking, but it's too high in fat to be part of a regular diet. Prepare it this way and you'll have all of the flavor of fried chicken without all of the extra fat.

2 teaspoons kosher salt

2 teaspoons fresh black pepper

6 skinless, boneless chicken breasts

2 cups plain nonfat yogurt

2 cups Special K cereal, crushed with a rolling pin or in a food
   processor or coffee grinder

Nonstick cooking spray

1. Preheat the oven to 375.

2. In a large plastic bag, combine the thyme, oregano, basil, garlic powder, salt, and pepper. Shake well. Add two breasts at a time to the bag and shake to coat the chicken. Continue until all the breasts are coated.

3. Place the yogurt in a large bowl, and the cereal on a large plate. Dip each breast in the yogurt and then in the cereal. Place the chicken breasts on a baking sheet sprayed with nonstick cooking spray.

4. Bake for 35 to 45 minutes, until the chicken is brown and cooked through. Do not cover or turn the chicken during the baking process.

5. When the chicken is completely cooked, remove the baking sheet from the oven and let cool 10 minutes before serving.

**NUTRITIONAL INFORMATION PER SERVING**
227 CALORIES · 32G PROTEIN · 4G FAT · 194MG SODIUM

# Curried Chicken

Many people have made a conscious decision to eat less red meat and more poultry in an effort to lower the fat in their diets. Light-meat chicken without the skin is up to 80 percent leaner than beef. And chicken breast is the leanest part of the chicken. That's one reason why I include this recipe in my book. The other reason is to illustrate the connection between soul food and Caribbean influence in some of my dishes.  *Serves 4*

¼ cup olive oil

1 garlic clove, minced

1 onion, cut into small dice

3 celery stalks, cut into small dice

4 scallions, sliced

1 pound skinless, boneless chicken breasts,
   cut into strips

4 tablespoons curry powder

2 teaspoons kosher salt

1 teaspoon fresh black pepper

1 cup chicken stock

1. Heat the oil in a medium-sized pot over high heat. Add the garlic, onion, celery, and scallions. Cook 3 to 5 minutes, or until the vegetables are soft.
2. Stir in the chicken, curry powder, salt, and pepper until well combined.
3. Add the stock and stir again. Bring to a boil. Reduce the heat and simmer for 25 to 30 minutes, until the chicken is cooked through and the sauce has thickened slightly.

**NUTRITIONAL INFORMATION PER SERVING**

387 CALORIES • 29G PROTEIN • 18G FAT • 308MG SODIUM

## Pineapple Barbecued Chicken

Although this recipe doesn't call for an actual barbecue, it's created in the great Southern tradition. Throughout the South, barbecue is an icon and a legacy, and many of the local and family barbecue recipes are guarded like jewels. *Serves 4*

2 cups olive oil

1 small onion, chopped

3 garlic cloves, minced

1 red pepper, cut into small dice

1 orange pepper, cut into small dice

2 carrots, peeled and cut into small dice

1 cup tomato sauce

2 cups honey

2 teaspoons peeled and minced ginger

2 teaspoons paprika

2 teaspoons kosher salt

2 teaspoons fresh black pepper

2 tablespoons brown sugar, firmly packed

1 pound skinless, boneless chicken breasts cut into strips

1 cup fresh pineapple chunks

1 cup Easy Vegetable Stock (page 68)

1. In a large pot, heat the oil over high heat. Add the onion and garlic and cook until soft.

2. Add the red and orange peppers, carrots, tomato sauce, honey, ginger, paprika, salt, black pepper, and brown sugar. Stir and cook for about 12 minutes, until the vegetables begin to soften and spice scents are released.

3. Combine the chicken with the vegetables and continue cooking for about 7 minutes, until the juices are released.

4. Add the pineapple and the stock and bring to a boil. Reduce the heat and simmer until the pineapple has softened, the chicken is cooked through, and the juices have reduced by half.

**NUTRITIONAL INFORMATION PER SERVING**

260 CALORIES · 21G PROTEIN · 5G FAT · 312MG SODIUM

# Lindsey's Peach Chicken

*Neo Soul* is about making soul food healthier without losing any of the tradition or flavor, and Lindsey's Peach Chicken is one of my special creations. I eat it at least once a week. The boiled-down peaches in this recipe add a tangy taste to this very healthy traditional chicken dish.

*Serves 6*

1 whole chicken, skinned, giblet bag removed

1 teaspoon Mrs. Dash seasoning blend

1 teaspoon kosher salt

1 teaspoon fresh black pepper

¼ cup olive oil

1 small onion, chopped

2 garlic cloves, minced

1 pound fresh peaches, peeled, pitted,
   and cut into eighths

2 cups chicken stock

1. Season the entire chicken inside and out with Mrs. Dash, salt, and pepper. Set aside.
2. Add the oil to a large braising pot and place over high heat. Add the onion and garlic and cook until soft—about 2 to 3 minutes. Add the chicken and brown on all sides. Remove the chicken and place on a plate.
3. Add the peaches to the pot and cook until they begin to soften and release their juices. Remove from the pot and place in a bowl.

4. Return the chicken to the pot and pour the peaches over it. Add the chicken stock, cover, and cook for 45 minutes to 1 hour, until the peaches are completely soft and the chicken is cooked thoroughly.

TIP: You might want to use a meat thermometer for this dish (and all the chicken dishes). Judging doneness on chicken can be tricky. A fully cooked chicken should register between 165 and 185 degrees when a thermometer inserted in the breast is read.

### NUTRITIONAL INFORMATION PER SERVING
326 CALORIES · 21G PROTEIN · 24G FAT · 64MG SODIUM

# Herb-Roasted Duck

There's an interesting combination of herbs used in this recipe. They flavor the meat and will make your kitchen smell wonderful. *Serves 8*

1 (5-pound) duck, whole, washed and dried, giblet bag removed

1½ cups olive oil

2 cups balsamic vinegar

2 teaspoons fresh black pepper

2 teaspoons chopped fresh rosemary leaves

2 teaspoons chopped fresh thyme leaves

1. In a nonreactive pan, marinate the duck in a mixture of the oil and the vinegar. Make sure that the marinade is on the inside as well as the outside of the duck. Marinate for 1 hour.
2. Preheat the oven to 375 degrees.
3. Transfer the duck to an oven-ready pan, if needed. Sprinkle the duck with the pepper, rosemary, and thyme on both on the inside and the outside and roast for 1 hour.

TIP: Be careful when cooking duck, especially whole duck. The fat that drips off of it is highly flammable! You may want to use a roasting rack and put some water in the bottom of the pan. The water will also help with the beginnings of a nice pan gravy.

**NUTRITIONAL INFORMATION PER SERVING**

720 CALORIES • 35G PROTEIN • 62G FAT • 114MG SODIUM

## Turkey Meatloaf

I've learned that using turkey instead of beef is a simple way to make your diet a little healthier and lower in fat. In this classic meatloaf, turkey is the way to go! *Serves 4*

1 pound ground turkey
2 cups finely diced red pepper
1 small onion, cut into small dice

1 cup fresh breadcrumbs

4 egg whites

1 teaspoon Mrs. Dash seasoning blend

1 garlic clove, minced

3 sprigs fresh thyme, stripped (leaves only) (see page 33)

1 tablespoon finely chopped fresh parsley leaves

2 cups tomato sauce

1. Preheat the oven to 350 degrees.
2. In a large bowl, combine all the ingredients and mix well. Use your hands to ensure that everything is evenly distributed. Form the mixture into a loaf and place it on the broiler pan.
3. Bake for 1 to 1½ hours. After the first hour, check every 15 minutes until evenly browned.
4. Remove the meatloaf from the oven and let it rest for 10 to 15 minutes before slicing.

**NUTRITIONAL INFORMATION PER SERVING**

89 CALORIES · 66G PROTEIN · 33G FAT · 90MG SODIUM

# Turkey Croquettes

You probably have a recipe or two for croquettes (what family doesn't?). Try this one next time and you'll be enjoying one of the favorite items from my celebrity catering menu. *Serves 4*

2 cups ground turkey, sautéed until no longer red

1 small onion, chopped

2 red peppers, minced

4 egg whites

⅛ teaspoon cayenne pepper

⅛ teaspoon garlic powder

Nonstick cooking spray

1. In a large bowl, combine all the ingredients except the cooking spray until they are well blended and the mixture holds together.
2. Using a ¼-cup measure, form the mixture into small balls and flatten slightly with your hand.
3. Spray a large skillet with nonstick cooking spray and place the skillet over medium heat. Place the croquettes in the heated skillet and cook for 3 to 4 minutes per side, until both sides are golden brown.

**NUTRITIONAL INFORMATION PER SERVING**

311 CALORIES · 30G PROTEIN · 24G FAT · 199MG SODIUM

## Grandma's Thanksgiving Turkey

Grandma Sylvia is famous for her turkey. On Thanksgiving each year, she prepares anywhere from 50 to 100 turkeys at the restaurant. I've made some changes to her more traditional recipe to make it even healthier, but the great flavor and accents are still here.    *Serves 24*

1 tablespoon Mrs. Dash
   seasoning blend

2 teaspoons fresh black pepper

2 teaspoons garlic powder

1 teaspoon kosher salt

1 (12-pound) turkey, washed and
   dried, giblet bag removed

4 sticks butter, at room temperature

4 cups turkey stock

6 tablespoons whole-wheat flour

1. In a small bowl, mix together the Mrs. Dash, black pepper, garlic powder, and salt. Sprinkle on top and inside the turkey. Cover with plastic wrap and let stand for 1 hour.
2. Preheat the oven to 350 degrees.
3. Prepare the roasting pan by covering the bottom with the butter. Place the turkey in the pan.
4. Cook for 1 hour. Then baste the bird and add 1 cup of the stock to the pan juices. Continue cooking another hour. Again baste, add ½ cup of stock, and baste again. Repeat for the third hour, remembering to baste and add water if needed.
5. The turkey will be completely cooked when the meat thermometer inserted in the breast shows a temperature of 170 degrees. (Either the thermometer provided in the turkey will pop or you can check to be sure with your own.)
6. Remove the pan from the oven and let cool for about 30 minutes.
7. Remove the bird from the pan. Then place the pan on the stove over medium heat, stirring constantly. Add the whole-wheat flour and 2 cups of stock to the pan and continue to stir. Cook until the mixture thickens and serve as gravy with the turkey.

**NUTRITIONAL INFORMATION PER SERVING**

568 CALORIES · 58G PROTEIN · 35G FAT · 150MG SODIUM

# Kenneth's Short Ribs of Beef

My mom's brother Kenneth is a huge fan of short ribs, and this recipe has been named in his honor. *Serves 6*

6 pieces beef short ribs, braised and cut to 1-inch thickness
1 teaspoon Mrs. Dash seasoning blend
2 teaspoons fresh black pepper
2 teaspoons garlic salt
¼ cup balsamic vinegar

1. Preheat the oven to 350 degrees.
2. Place the beef in a baking dish.
3. In a small bowl, combine the Mrs. Dash, black pepper, and garlic salt. Sprinkle the mixture all over the short ribs. Pour the vinegar over the beef and marinate for 1 hour.
4. Place the marinated beef in a casserole or similar type dish with a cover. Cook covered for 45 minutes. Remove the cover and cook an additional 15 minutes. Let cool and serve.

NUTRITIONAL INFORMATION PER SERVING

309 CALORIES • 17G PROTEIN • 24G FAT • 63MG SODIUM

# Beef Stew

~~~~~~~~

Here's a hearty and satisfying comfort food that's a healthy meal, too.

*Serves 8*

¼ cup olive oil

2 onions, cut into small dice

1 garlic clove, minced

2 pounds 95% lean beef, cut
   into cubes

½ cup flour

1 red pepper, cut into small
   dice

1 yellow pepper, cut into
   small dice

4 carrots, peeled and cut
   into small dice

¼ cup soy sauce

1 cup beef stock

2 teaspoons fresh black
   pepper

1. Heat the oil in a large pot over high heat. Add the onions and garlic and cook until they begin to brown.
2. Lightly dust the beef cubes with the flour and add them to the pot. Continue cooking until the beef begins to brown and release its juices, about 8 to 10 minutes.
3. Stir in the red and yellow peppers and the carrot. Add the soy sauce, beef stock, and black pepper. Bring the stew to a boil.
4. Reduce the heat and simmer for 30 to 40 minutes, until the beef is tender and the sauce has thickened.

**NUTRITIONAL INFORMATION PER SERVING**

420 CALORIES · 32G PROTEIN · 26G FAT · 594MG SODIUM

# Marinated Roast Beef with Roasted Squash and Vegetables

~~~~~~~~~~~~~~~~~~~~~~~~~~~~

A recent survey revealed that 85 percent of consumers are not eating the recommended minimum of five servings of produce per day. This great meal includes three vegetables as well as delicious roast beef.

*Serves 10*

1 (3-pound) beef roast, trimmed and tied

¼ cup Mrs. Dash seasoning blend

2 teaspoons kosher salt

2 teaspoons fresh black pepper

2 cups olive oil

1 butternut squash, peeled, seeded, and cubed

3 carrots, peeled and cut into large dice

2 celery stalks, cut into large dice

1. Preheat the oven to 350 degrees.
2. In a medium bowl, combine the Mrs. Dash, 1 teaspoon of the salt, 1 teaspoon of the pepper, and 1 cup of the oil. Cover the beef with the oil mixture and let it marinate for 1 hour at room temperature.
3. Place the squash, carrots, and celery in a large bowl. Combine the remaining oil, salt, and pepper and let the vegetables marinate in this mixture.
4. Place the roast in a large baking dish and arrange the vegetables around it. Bake for 1 to 1½ hours. Cut the meat in the center to check for desired doneness.

5. When completely cooked, remove the beef from the oven and let it rest for at least 20 minutes before cutting.
6. Arrange the vegetables around the beef to serve.

### NUTRITIONAL INFORMATION PER SERVING
371 CALORIES · 38G PROTEIN · 67G FAT · 290MG SODIUM

# Sunday Chuck Roast

In our family, as in most traditional Southern families, Sunday dinner starts early and lasts for hours. Chuck roast is a hearty dish that remains a staple in many of our Sunday dinners. *Serves 8*

1 (3-pound) chuck roast
1 teaspoon kosher salt
1 teaspoon fresh black pepper
4 carrots, peeled and cut into large dice
3 Idaho potatoes, peeled and cut into large dice
2 large onions, peeled and quartered
2 cups beef stock

1. Preheat the oven to 300 degrees.
2. Season the roast with salt and pepper and place in a shallow baking dish. Arrange the carrots, potatoes, and onions around the meat. Sprinkle with the stock and cover with aluminum foil.

3. Bake for 3½ to 4 hours, or until the meat is tender when pierced with a fork.

TIP: Minimal seasoning is fine with this cut of meat. There is so much natural flavor released during the cooking process that no additional seasoning is needed.

NUTRITIONAL INFORMATION PER SERVING

588 CALORIES · 41G PROTEIN · 49G FAT · 12MG SODIUM

6

# Desserts

When I was young, I loved dessert. Grandma Julia was an amazing baker. Her sweet potato pies, coconut pies, and pound cakes are still the best I've ever had. I know they inspired my Grandma Sylvia's recipes at the restaurant.

But for people with a food addiction, desserts can be dangerous territory. You really have to know yourself when it comes to your desserts. For instance, it's definitely not a good idea to eat your meals with the sole purpose of getting to dessert! This chapter is filled with healthy, flavorful desserts that won't make you feel deprived when others are eating theirs.

Personally, I prefer having fruit for dessert, mixed with yogurt and a little bit of sugar. I particularly like strawberries—they seem like a dessert fruit. But I rarely eat flour or sugar, simply because I don't want to get used to knowing I can have those ingredients. When you're addicted to

flour and sugar, as I was, then it's generally not a good idea to experiment, even with healthy recipes.

And for those of you who are trying to reduce your weight without
necessarily battling a food addiction, this section will show you how to
feed your sweet tooth without all the sugar and calories of traditional
desserts.

## Banana Pound Cake

In the South, pound cake is part of a long tradition, especially at Christ-
mastime. I know my great-grandmother Julia, a pound cake lover, would
have approved of this recipe.

Although this cake can be eaten immediately, the flavor does improve
with time. Make 24 hours ahead for maximum taste.    *Serves 12*

Nonstick cooking spray
4½ cups whole-wheat or unbleached flour
4 sticks butter
2 cups sugar
2 cups egg whites
5 medium bananas, peeled and well mashed

1. Preheat the oven to 350 degrees. Spray a 10-inch round cake pan with
   nonstick cooking spray and dust with flour. Set aside.

2. Using the paddle attachment of a mixer, cream the butter and sugar together until they are well combined and have a uniform consistency.

3. Add the egg whites slowly, in stages, being sure to mix between each addition, until all the egg whites are absorbed.

4. Add 2 cups of the flour. Mix well until all the flour is absorbed. Add the bananas and mix until combined. Add the remaining 2½ cups flour and continue to mix until the entire mixture is well beaten. Pour the batter into the prepared cake pan.

5. Bake for about 1 hour, or until the crack in the top is brown and shows no moistness. Or you can insert a toothpick into the center of the cake; if the toothpick comes out clean, the cake is done (see box below).

6. Let the cake cool in its pan on a cake rack for 5 minutes, then remove it from the pan and let it continue to cool directly on the rack.

**NUTRITIONAL INFORMATION PER SERVING**

620 CALORIES · 11G PROTEIN · 33G FAT · 72MG SODIUM

## · TOOTHPICK TEST ·

Most cooks know this baking tip, but it's worth repeating for the newer chefs. The "clean toothpick test" is used in baking to determine "doneness." Insert a clean, dry toothpick into the center of the item you are baking. If the pick is clean when pulled out, the item is cooked thoroughly.

# Apple Crisp

~~~~~~~~~

Crisps are part of our dessert tradition. You can try this recipe with a different type of fruit. For example, you could use peaches, pears, or cherries for a delightful crisp.   *Serves 8*

Nonstick cooking spray
10 Granny Smith apples, cored, peeled, and sliced
3 tablespoons fresh lemon juice
¼ cup apple cider
1 cup whole-wheat or unbleached flour
2 cups rolled oats
1 cup brown sugar, firmly packed
1 tablespoon ground cinnamon
1 teaspoon kosher salt
1 stick butter, at room temperature

1. Preheat the oven to 350 degrees. Spray a 9x13-inch baking dish with nonstick cooking spray and lay the apple slices in the bottom.
2. In a small bowl, combine the lemon juice and cider. Pour the mixture over the apples.
3. In a medium-sized bowl, combine the flour, oats, brown sugar, cinnamon, and salt. Mix until combined. Rub the butter into the dry ingredients with your hands until the mixture resembles coarse crumbs. Spread the mixture over the apples to cover them.
4. Bake for 45 minutes, or until the apples are soft. Remove the baking dish from the oven, let cool, and serve.

TIP: Use your favorite variety of apple when making this crisp. Just remember that a harder or crisper apple may require you to lengthen the cooking time. Granny Smith apples work best for the cooking time suggested in this recipe.

NUTRITIONAL INFORMATION PER SERVING

261 CALORIES  •  6G PROTEIN  •  11G FAT  •  13MG SODIUM

## Bread Pudding

Bread pudding is a special treat that should be enjoyed in small portions.

*Serves 12*

¼ teaspoon butter

6 eggs

2 cups sugar

1 quart half-and-half

¼ cup pure vanilla extract

1-pound loaf of day-old bread, sliced, buttered on one side,
    and cubed

1. Preheat the oven to 300 degrees. Butter a 9x12-inch baking dish or similar dish with the ¼ teaspoon butter.
2. In a large bowl, beat the eggs and sugar together. Add the half-and-half and then the vanilla. Continue to beat until well combined. The mixture should resemble custard.

3. Place the bread in the baking dish and pour the custard mixture over it.
4. Bake for about 40 minutes.

VARIATION: Try adding your favorite dried or fresh fruit to this recipe. Just before baking, sprinkle the pudding with blueberries, raisins, fresh or dried currants, or sliced peaches or apricots. Create your own classic!

NUTRITIONAL INFORMATION PER SERVING

287 CALORIES • 8G PROTEIN • 13G FAT • 267MG SODIUM

# Pineapple Upside-Down Cake

Every Southern family has a recipe for pineapple upside-down cake. Like so many other dessert favorites, this is rich and filled with calories, so just have one small piece. I no longer eat pineapple upside-down cake, but I remember as a kid licking the bowls, licking my fingers, and asking for seconds. *Serves 12*

CAKE:

Butter for coating pan
3 eggs, separated
1 cup sugar
1 cup canned or fresh pineapple juice
1 cup flour

1 teaspoon baking powder

⅛ teaspoon kosher salt

Topping:

1 stick butter

1 cup brown sugar, firmly packed

1 (16-ounce) can sliced pineapple, or 1 medium pineapple, cored
  and sliced into rounds

2 tablespoons whole pecans

1. Preheat the oven to 375 degrees. Generously coat a 10-inch tube pan with butter.

2. In a large bowl, begin preparing the cake batter by beating the egg yolks until light in color. Beat together with the sugar.

3. Add the pineapple juice, flour, baking powder, and salt. Mix until well combined and set.

4. In a medium-sized bowl, beat the egg whites until they form stiff peaks. Fold into the batter and set aside.

5. To make the topping, melt the 1 stick butter in a small saucepan. Pour it into the buttered tube pan. Spread the brown sugar evenly over the bottom of the pan. Arrange the pineapple slices on the brown sugar, then drop the pecans in the empty spaces.

6. Cover it all with the cake batter.

7. Bake about 30 minutes, or until a toothpick inserted in the center comes out clean. When it's done, place a large plate over the pan and turn the cake over onto the plate to cool.

NUTRITIONAL INFORMATION PER SERVING

257 CALORIES  ·  3G PROTEIN  ·  10G FAT  ·  126MG SODIUM

# Fried Apples

~~~~~~~~~~~~~

To make these fried apples even healthier, cut the flour and sugar amounts in this recipe in half, and lightly fry the apples in half the amount of oil.   *Serves 10*

| | |
|---|---|
| 1 cup flour | 3 cups vegetable oil |
| 1 teaspoon sugar | 10 apples, cored and sliced |
| ½ teaspoon kosher salt |    (peeled or unpeeled) |
| ⅔ cup skim or lowfat milk |    (use your favorite variety) |
| 2 eggs, well beaten | Dash confectioners' sugar |

1. In a large bowl, whisk together the flour, sugar, and salt until combined. Slowly add the milk, then gradually mix in the eggs. Continue to whisk the batter.
2. In a large skillet, heat about 2 inches of oil over high heat.
3. Dust the apples lightly with flour, dip them in the batter, and gently place them in the hot oil. Cook the apples, in batches (be sure not to crowd the pot), for about 4 minutes, or until they are golden brown. Feel free to adjust the cooking time if the color is too light or too dark.
4. Remove the apples from the skillet and drain on a paper towel–lined plate. Sprinkle with confectioners' sugar and serve.

**NUTRITIONAL INFORMATION PER SERVING**

292 CALORIES · 3G PROTEIN · 13G FAT · 111MG SODIUM

# Peach Cobbler

~~~~~~~~~~~~~~~~

You don't have to be from the South to make the best peach cobbler in the world—but it helps. As a kid, I would pick the peaches right off the tree, deliver them to my grandmother, and watch her prepare a cobbler like this one. Once again, prepare desserts sensibly and eat them sparingly, and you can enjoy an occasional treat without ruining your healthful diet. *Serves 10*

1¾ cup flour
⅓ cup brown sugar, firmly packed
1 tablespoon baking powder
1 teaspoon cinnamon
½ teaspoon kosher salt
½ teaspoon grated nutmeg
¼ teaspoon allspice
1 stick butter
1 cup skim or lowfat milk
4 cups peaches, either 5 fresh peaches, peeled and sliced,
    or 3 (10-ounce) packages frozen peaches, thawed,
    drained, and sliced

1. Preheat the oven to 350 degrees.
2. In a large bowl, combine the flour, brown sugar, baking powder, cinnamon, salt, nutmeg, and allspice.

3. Cut in the butter until the mixture resembles small peas. Slowly add the milk.

4. Place the peaches in the bottom of a 9x12-inch baking dish. Pour the flour mixture evenly on top.

5. Bake for 35 to 45 minutes, until the top is brown and bubbly.

### NUTRITIONAL INFORMATION PER SERVING

277 CALORIES · 4G PROTEIN · 2G FAT · 212MG SODIUM

## Blueberry Buckle

Blueberry buckle is finger-lickin' good . . . if you like blueberries, as I do.

*Serves 10*

CAKE:

Nonstick cooking spray

2 cups flour

2 teaspoons baking powder

½ teaspoon kosher salt

¾ cup sugar

½ stick butter, at room temperature

1 egg

½ cup skim or lowfat milk

2 cups fresh blueberries or frozen, thawed,
    and drained

STREUSEL TOPPING:

½ cup sugar

⅓ cup flour

½ teaspoon cinnamon

¼ stick butter, at room temperature

1. Preheat the oven to 350 degrees. Spray a 9x9-inch square baking dish with nonstick cooking spray.
2. In a large bowl, combine the 2 cups flour and the baking powder and salt. Whisk together well and set aside.
3. In a small bowl, combine the ¾ cup sugar, the ½ stick butter, and the egg and milk. Stir until well combined and set aside.
4. Lightly dust the blueberries with flour. Remove excess by shaking the berries in a colander.
5. Add the egg mixture to the dry mixture. Combine well and then fold in the blueberries. Set aside.
6. To make the topping, combine the ½ cup sugar, the ⅓ cup flour, the cinnamon, and the ¼ stick butter in a small bowl. Use a fork to blend until it looks like wet sand.
7. Pour the blueberry mixture into the prepared baking dish. Top with the streusel and bake for about 40 minutes, until golden brown. Remove from the oven and let cool slightly. Serve slightly warm.

NUTRITIONAL INFORMATION PER SERVING

266 CALORIES · 4G PROTEIN · 9G FAT · 88MG SODIUM

# Pumpkin Pie

Cakes and pies of all types are part of my family's holiday celebrations. Pumpkin pie remains a true classic and a family favorite.    *Serves 12*

PASTRY (MAKES 2 CRUSTS):

8 ounces cream cheese

2 sticks butter, at room temperature

2 cups flour

FILLING:

½ stick butter

3 tablespoons brown sugar, firmly packed

1 medium pumpkin, washed, halved, and seeded

1 cup water, more or less

2 tablespoons cinnamon

1 tablespoon grated nutmeg

1 tablespoon ground ginger

1 tablespoon ground clove

2 eggs

1 (14-ounce) can sweetened condensed milk

1. To make the pastry, cream together the cream cheese and the 2 sticks butter in a large bowl until smooth. Add the flour and stir until the mixture forms a dough ball. Divide the pastry mixture in half and wrap each half in plastic wrap. Pound each into a disk and chill for at least 1 hour.

2. To make the filling, melt the ½ stick butter and brown sugar in a small saucepan. Let cool slightly.

3. Coat the pumpkin halves with the brown sugar mixture, place them cut side down on a baking sheet, and roast in the oven until soft and collapsed.

4. Remove the pumpkin from the oven and let cool. With a large spoon, scoop out the flesh and blend in a food processor. Thin the mixture out by adding any drippings left in the pan. Continue blending, adding water gradually until a "thick batter" consistency is reached. Place the mixture in a bowl. Add the cinnamon, nutmeg, ginger, and clove and stir until well combined.

5. Measure out 2 cups of batter and place in a large bowl. Add the eggs and condensed milk. Whisk together well and set aside.

6. Preheat the oven to 350 degrees.

7. Remove one dough disk and roll out to a 9-inch circle. Line a pie plate with the crust, secure the edges, and fill with the filling to the top.

8. Bake for 30 to 45 minutes, until the filling "domes" in the center. Remove and let cool.

**NUTRITIONAL INFORMATION PER SERVING**

500 CALORIES · 9G PROTEIN · 15G FAT · 314MG SODIUM

# Coconut Cake

〜〜〜〜〜〜〜

Coconut milk is such a healthy drink that many families feed it to their infants. Like so many other desserts, coconut cake is filled with things that are good for you, plus some ingredients you want to take in moderation. There wasn't one family holiday or celebration that didn't include this dessert. *Serves 16*

CAKE:

1 large fresh coconut

3 eggs, separated

1½ cups sugar

1½ sticks butter

½ teaspoon pure vanilla extract

2¼ cups sifted cake flour

2¼ teaspoons baking powder

½ teaspoon kosher salt

4 to 6 tablespoons skim or lowfat milk,
    if needed


FROSTING:

2 cups sugar

1 (12-ounce) can evaporated milk

1 stick butter

1 teaspoon pure vanilla extract

1 large fresh coconut, grated

1. To begin making the cake, grate the coconut, reserving the coconut milk. Preheat the oven to 350 degrees.

2. Beat the egg whites to soft peaks, while gradually adding ½ cup of the sugar. Set aside.

3. In a separate bowl, beat the egg yolks until thick. Set aside.

4. Cream the 1½ sticks butter with the ½ teaspoon vanilla in a large bowl. Beat in the remaining 1 cup sugar. Stir the egg yolks into the butter mixture and cream well. Set aside.

5. Sift the sifted flour, baking powder, and salt together three times.

6. Add enough milk to the reserved coconut milk to make 1 cup liquid. Alternate adding the milk mixture and the flour mixture to the butter mixture. Blend in ¼ cup of the grated coconut (reserving ¾ cup for sprinkling the finished cake) and beat well. Fold in the egg whites.

7. Pour into two 9-inch or three 8-inch layer pans. Bake for 25 to 30 minutes, until golden brown and a toothpick inserted in the center comes out clean.

8. To make the frosting, combine the 2 cups sugar, the evaporated milk, the 1 stick butter, and the 1 teaspoon vanilla in a saucepan and cook for about 5 minutes on low to medium heat, until the mixture begins to thicken. Mix in the coconut.

9. Frost the cake layers, assemble, and sprinkle with the remaining grated coconut.

NUTRITIONAL INFORMATION PER SERVING

649 CALORIES · 7G PROTEIN · 40G FAT · 54MG SODIUM

# Chocolate Cake with Chocolate Frosting

Well, there's not much I can do with a traditional chocolate cake recipe to make it totally healthy and good for you, so just limit yourself to one small piece if you are trying to eat healthy. If you have a craving for a delicious chocolate cake, I guarantee you will love this one. *Serves 12*

CAKE:

¾ cup sugar

½ cup flour

¼ teaspoon baking soda

⅛ teaspoon kosher salt

¼ cup unsweetened cocoa powder

¼ cup boiling water

⅓ cup applesauce

¼ cup egg substitute

1 teaspoon pure vanilla extract

FROSTING:

8 ounces light cream cheese

1 tablespoon butter

2 cups Splenda

½ cup unsweetened cocoa powder

⅛ teaspoon kosher salt

1 teaspoon pure vanilla extract

3 tablespoons skim milk, if needed

1. Preheat the oven to 350 degrees. Line an 8-inch cake pan with a circle of baking parchment cut to fit the bottom of the pan.

2. In a large bowl, mix the sugar, flour, baking soda, and ⅛ teaspoon salt. Dissolve the ¼ cup cocoa powder in the boiling water and then add to the dry ingredients. Mix well.

3. Stir in the applesauce, egg substitute, and 1 teaspoon vanilla. Pour the batter into the prepared pan. Bake for 35 minutes.

4. To make the frosting, beat the cream cheese and butter with an electric mixer until smooth. Add the Splenda and beat until incorporated. Add the ½ cup cocoa powder, ⅛ teaspoon salt, and 1 teaspoon vanilla and beat until blended. If the frosting is too thick to spread, add the milk, 1 tablespoon at a time, with the mixer on low, until spreading consistency is achieved. Let the cake cool completely on a cooling rack before frosting.

**NUTRITIONAL INFORMATION PER SERVING**

357 CALORIES · 5G PROTEIN · 7G FAT · 230MG SODIUM

# Old-Fashioned Apple Pie

There's really no dish as American as apple pie. In the South, pies of all sorts are part of the great dessert tradition in every family. Apple pie is good fresh out of the oven, and even better the next day. Two of the younger members of my family, Macali and Zaire, are carrying on the great apple pie tradition in our family by baking them for special family get-togethers. *Serves 12*

PASTRY:

8 ounces cream cheese

2 sticks butter, at room temperature

2 cups flour

FILLING:

1 tablespoon flour

⅔ cup sugar (you might need more or less, depending on the
   sweetness of the apples used)

¼ teaspoon cinnamon

8 apples, cored, peeled, and sliced evenly (use your
   favorite variety)

1 tablespoon butter

½ teaspoon fresh lemon juice

1 egg, beaten

1. Preheat the oven to 450 degrees.
2. To make the pastry, cream together the cream cheese and 2 sticks but-

ter in a large bowl until smooth. Add the 2 cups flour and stir until the mixture forms a dough ball. Divide the pastry mixture in half and wrap each half in plastic wrap. Pound each half into a disk and chill for at least 1 hour.

3. Roll out one disk to a 9-inch circle and line a 9-inch pie pan with the pastry, fitting carefully into edges. Set aside.

4. To make the filling, combine the 1 tablespoon flour, the sugar, and cinnamon in a small bowl. Place one layer of apples on the bottom of the pan and sprinkle with half of the sugar mixture. Arrange another layer of apples and sprinkle with the remaining mixture. Dot the top with the 1 tablespoon butter and sprinkle with the lemon juice.

5. Roll out the other disk of pastry. Brush the edges of the lower crust with the beaten egg, lay the top crust on top of the filling, and seal the upper and lower crusts together. Trim the excess and flute (crimp the finished edge) if desired. With a sharp knife, cut random steam vents in the top pastry.

6. Bake in the 450-degree oven for 15 minutes, then reduce the heat to 325 degrees and bake for an additional 35 to 40 minutes, until the apples are well cooked and the crust is a golden brown.

7. Let cool to lukewarm before cutting.

### NUTRITIONAL INFORMATION PER SERVING
455 CALORIES • 5G PROTEIN • 25G FAT • 170MG SODIUM

# Pecan Pie

~~~~~~~~~~

There was a big old pecan tree in my grandmother's front yard in South Carolina. As a boy I would climb that tree, knock down the pecans, open them up, and beg Grandma to make me a pecan pie.   *Serves 12*

PASTRY:

4 ounces cream cheese

1 stick butter, at room temperature

1 cup flour

FILLING:

1 cup sugar

½ stick butter

¼ teaspoon kosher salt

6 eggs

1¼ cups dark corn syrup

1½ teaspoons pure vanilla extract

5 ounces pecan quarters

1. To make the pastry, cream the cream cheese and the 1 cup butter in a large bowl until smooth. Add the flour and stir until the mixture forms a dough ball. Wrap pastry mixture in plastic wrap. Pound into a disk and chill for at least 1 hour.

2. Preheat the oven to 450 degrees.

3. To make the filling, select the paddle attachment of the mixer and on low speed blend the sugar, ½ stick butter, and salt well. While the

machine is running, add the eggs, one at a time, until absorbed. Add the syrup and vanilla and mix until well blended. Set aside.

4. Roll out one 9-inch bottom pastry. Place in the pie dish and carefully press into place. Evenly distribute the pecans on the crust. Fill with the sugar mixture.

5. Bake at 450 for 10 minutes. Reduce the heat to 350 and bake about 40 minutes more. Remove and let cool.

**NUTRITIONAL INFORMATION PER SERVING**

464 CALORIES · 6G PROTEIN · 31G FAT · 372MG SODIUM

# Red Velvet Cake

This cake, when done well, is just beautiful to look at and even better to taste! It's flavored with chocolate and cream cheese frosting and should be considered a special treat. My editor insisted on including **Red Velvet Cake** in *Neo Soul*. This recipe is probably healthier than the one your grandmother used—and tastes just as good.    *Serves 12*

2 sticks unsalted butter, at room temperature

1½ cups sifted cake flour

1½ cups granulated sugar

2 eggs

2 teaspoons unsweetened cocoa powder

2 ounces red food coloring

1 teaspoon salt

1 teaspoon pure vanilla extract

1 cup buttermilk

1½ teaspoons white vinegar

1 teaspoon baking soda

FROSTING:

16 ounces cream cheese, at room temperature

1 stick unsalted butter, at room temperature

2 pounds confectioners' sugar

1 teaspoon pure vanilla extract

1. Preheat the oven to 350 degrees. Grease with butter and flour two 9-inch cake pans. Cut out two 9-inch round pieces of baking parchment paper and grease and flour the paper. Place one on the bottom of each cake pan.

2. Cream the 2 sticks butter, the granulated sugar, and the eggs in a heavy-duty mixer.

3. In a small bowl, combine the cocoa and food coloring and add to the butter mixture.

4. Mix the salt and 1 teaspoon vanilla with the buttermilk in a 2-cup liquid measuring cup. Alternately, add the butter mixture and the buttermilk mixture to the flour, a little at a time.

5. Mix the vinegar and baking soda in a small bowl (this will fizz). Carefully and gently fold this into the batter. *Do not beat!*

6. Divide the batter between the cake pans and bake for 30 minutes, or until the cake layers spring back when lightly touched. Remove from the oven and let cool on racks for 15 minutes. Invert the cakes onto the racks, remove the parchment, and let cool to room temperature.

7. To make the frosting, beat the cream cheese and 1 stick butter together in a heavy-duty mixer until smooth and creamy.

8. Slowly add the confectioners' sugar, ½ cup at a time, blending after each addition. Mix in the 1 teaspoon vanilla. Beat for about 5 minutes until very smooth.

9. Frost the layers and carefully stack the cake.

### NUTRITIONAL INFORMATION PER SERVING

419 CALORIES · 6G PROTEIN · 21G FAT · 289MG SODIUM

## Three-Way Pecan Pound Cake

There's a little more work involved in creating this cake than some others. "Three-way" refers to the three different mixtures you prepare and combine to get the actual cake batter.  *Serves 12*

3 sticks butter, at room temperature

½ cup brown sugar, firmly packed

1 pound pecans, chopped

3 cups white sugar

6 eggs, at room temperature

3 cups flour

¼ teaspoon salt

½ teaspoon baking powder

1 teaspoon pure vanilla extract

1 cup skim or lowfat milk

1. Preheat the oven to 350 degrees.

2. Heat 1 stick of the butter in a small saucepan. Add the brown sugar and ½ cup of the pecans. Set aside, but keep the pan warm.

3. With the paddle attachment of the mixer, beat the remaining 2 sticks butter and the white sugar until creamy. Add the eggs, one at a time, until the yolks disappear. Set the butter mixture aside.

4. Combine the flour, salt, and baking powder and 1 cup of the pecans in a large bowl. Set aside.

5. In a small bowl, stir the vanilla and the milk together.

6. Alternately add the flour mixture and the milk mixture to the butter mixture in small amounts. The final addition should be the flour mixture. This is the cake batter.

7. Grease with butter and flour a 10-inch tube pan. Spread the warm brown sugar mixture on the bottom of the pan. Pour the cake batter over the brown sugar mixture. Shake or firmly set the pan on the counter to release air bubbles. Sprinkle the top with pecans to taste.

8. Bake for 1 hour and 15 minutes, or until a toothpick inserted in the center comes out clean. Let the cake cool in the pan on a wire rack for 10 to 15 minutes. Remove the cake from the pan and let cool completely on the rack.

NUTRITIONAL INFORMATION PER SERVING

850 CALORIES · 11G PROTEIN · 55G FAT · 370MG SODIUM

# Neo Sweet Potato Pie

~~~~~~~~~~~~~~~~~~~~~~~~~~~~~~

I grew up with sweet potatoes and yams as part of my family's cooking. One of my favorite soul food dishes has always been sweet potato pie.

*Serves 10*

2 sticks butter

2 cups honey

1 teaspoon cinnamon

1 teaspoon grated nutmeg

1 pound sweet potatoes, peeled and cut into chunks

2 eggs

1 (14-ounce) can sweetened condensed milk

1 9-inch whole-wheat pie shell

1. In a medium saucepan, melt the butter with the honey over low heat. Remove from the heat and whisk in the cinnamon and nutmeg. Set aside.

2. Place the sweet potatoes in a large bowl and toss with the butter mixture. Place in a baking dish and bake for 45 to 50 minutes, until the potatoes are very soft. Remove the dish from the oven and let cool.

3. Preheat the oven to 350 degrees.

4. In a large bowl, mash the cooked sweet potatoes with a potato masher, or you can use a food processor or hand blender. As you mash the potatoes, you can add water, a tablespoon at a time, to create a more liquid consistency. When the mixture is smooth and lump-free, mea-

sure out 2 cups and place in a medium bowl or a large measuring cup with a spout.

5.  In a small or medium bowl, whisk together the eggs and milk. Combine with the sweet potatoes and blend until mixed well. Pour into the pie shell.

6.  Bake for 40 minutes, or until the top begins to expand.

7.  Remove the shell from the oven and let cool. Slice and serve warm or at room temperature.

NUTRITIONAL INFORMATION PER SERVING

378 CALORIES · 8G PROTEIN · 52G FAT · 49MG SODIUM

# Index